The
Health Teacher's
BOOK of LISTS

PATRICIA RIZZO-TONER, M.Ed.
MARIAN D. MILLIKEN, M.Ed.

**THE CENTER FOR APPLIED RESEARCH
IN EDUCATION**

Library of Congress Cataloging-in-Publication Data

Toner, Patricia Rizzo
  The health teacher's book of lists / Patricia Rizzo Toner, Marian
D. Milliken.
      p.   cm.
    ISBN 0-87628-476-4
    1. Health education—United States—Handbooks, manuals, etc.
I. Milliken, Marian D.   II. Title.
LB1588.U6T66   1999
372.3'7—dc21   98–50233
                                                           CIP

Acquisitions Editor: *Connie Kallback*
Production Editor: *Tom Curtin*
Interior Design/Formatter: *Dee Coroneos*

© 1999 by The Center for Applied Research in Education, West Nyack, New York

Printed in the United States of America

10 9 8 7 6 5 4 3 2

ISBN 0-87628-476-4

ATTENTION: CORPORATIONS AND SCHOOLS

The Center for Applied Research in Education books are available at quantity discounts with bulk purchase for educational, business, or sales promotional use. For information, please write to: Prentice Hall Direct, Special Sales, 240 Frisch Court, Paramus, NJ 07652. Please supply: title of book, ISBN, quantity, how the book will be used, date needed.

**THE CENTER FOR APPLIED RESEARCH
IN EDUCATION**
West Nyack, NY 10994

www.phdirect.com

DEDICATION

This book is dedicated to my son, Dan Toner of Holland, Pennsylvania,
and
to administrators Dennis Warg and Dave Yates, Council Rock High School;
Sheila Murphy, Neshaminy High School; and Mark Collins, Holland Junior High
School; they have all provided much guidance and encouragement in both my
teaching and my coaching careers.

Patricia Rizzo-Toner

To the joys of my life, my children,
Lisa, Christy, and Troy.
You make up my most favorite list of them all.
I love you.

Marian D. Milliken

ACKNOWLEDGMENTS

Much of the clip art used throughout this book was from Nova Development Corporation's *Gold Edition ART EXPLOSION 125,000 Images,* copyright 1995-1996, which has proven to be an invaluable tool for desktop publishing.

For further information: http://www.novadevcorp.com.

Special thanks to:

My family—especially my son Dan—for providing love, encouragement, and support.

Steve Harnish, Council Rock High School, Newtown, Pennsylvania, for reviewing some of the material, and for being a dynamic and dedicated teacher and a very dear friend.

Connie Kallback and Win Huppuch of Prentice Hall for allowing me the freedom to try new ideas.

My assistant field hockey and lacrosse coaches, Gwen Davis and Terry Brookshaw, for your never-ending support, dedication, and friendship. I know I can ALWAYS count on you. Thank you.

Patricia Rizzo-Toner

To my family for providing me with encouragement, laughter, and love.

To my editor, Connie Kallback, for her generous guidance and insight.

To my friend, Pat Toner, for her patience, talent, humor, and friendship.

To my daughter, Christy McCall, for her endless research, proofreading, enthusiasm, and smile.

And to my students—each one of you—for all that you have taught me.

Thank you all. I am indeed fortunate to have you all in my life.

Marian D. Milliken

ABOUT THE AUTHORS

Patricia Rizzo-Toner, M.Ed., has taught health and physical education in the Council Rock School District, Newtown, PA, for over twenty-four years and coaches field hockey and lacrosse. She is the author or co-author of nine books including: Volumes 1-6: *Just for the HEALTH of it! Health Curriculum Activities Library (1993), What Are We Doing in Gym Today?, You'll Never Guess What We Did in Gym Today!, and How to Survive Teaching Health.* Besides her work as a teacher, guest speaker, and coach, Pat is a freelance cartoonist, a member of AAH-PERD, and was named to Who's Who Among Students in American Colleges and Universities, as well as Who's Who in American Education.

Marian Milliken, M.Ed., has taught health and physical education in the Council Rock School District, Newtown, PA, for over twenty years. She serves as advisor to over 900 students in the S.A.D.D. (Students Against Doing Drugs) chapter and is a member of the nationally recognized Student Assistance Team. In addition to her work as a teacher, Marian has coached field hockey and track. A member of AAHPERD, Marian received the Patricia Chamberlain Award for Excellence in the field of health and physical education and has recently been elected to Who's Who in American Education.

ABOUT THIS RESOURCE

The Health Teacher's Book of Lists is an all-in-one resource developed to give you—the busy classroom teacher—a wealth of ideas and information for planning lessons, discussions, projects, reports and activities in grades K–12. The nearly 300 basic and advanced lists, which you can reproduce for student use or keep on hand as a comprehensive reference tool, have been organized into fourteen main sections.

➡ **Section 1, Systems of the Body,** provides 25 lists on topics dealing with all of the body systems, such as "Major Skeletal Muscles, Muscle Types, and Their Functions" (7), "Main Divisions of the Brain" (10), "Functions and Structure of the Digestive System" (17), and "Interesting Facts About the Human Body" (25).

➡ **Section 2, Human Sexuality,** offers 20 basic-to-advanced lists including, "Male Physiology" (30), "Male Sexual Concerns" (34), "Organs of the Female Reproductive System" (internal and external—35, and 36), "Risk Factors for Breast Cancer" (40), and "Phases of Human Sexual Response" (44).

➡ **Section 3, Diet and Nutrition,** offers 21 lists, including "Essential Nutrients Found in Food" (46), "U.S. Recommended Daily Dietary Allowances" (55), "Common Causes of Overweight and Obesity" (61), and "Common Eating Disorders" (64).

➡ **Section 4, Consumer Health,** includes 17 lists, such as "Consumer Bill of Rights" (68), "Health Products Commonly Susceptible to Fraud" (71), "Guidelines for Choosing a Health Professional" (78), and "Questions to Ask About Prescription Drugs" (81).

➡ **Section 5, First Aid and Safety,** features 28 lists, for example, "Techniques to Control Severe Bleeding" (93), "Symptoms of and First Aid for Shock" (95), and other first-aid lists dealing with poisoning, weather-related emergencies, choking, broken bones, and sudden illness.

➡ **Section 6, Diseases and Disorders,** offers a comprehensive set of 21 lists, such as "Types of Pathogens and Ways They Can Be Spread" (113), "Types of Vaccines" (114), "Three Basic Defenses Against Infection" (122), and "Interesting Facts About Diseases and Disorders" (132).

➡ **Section 7, Sexually Transmitted Infections, HIV, and AIDS,** provides 17 lists on symptoms of STIs, HIV, and AIDS in general, as well as specific lists, such as "General Symptoms in Females" (134), "Risky Behaviors Known to Transmit HIV" (141), "HIV Diagnostic Tests" (145), and "Infections Included in the CDC's Definition of AIDS" (147).

➡ **Section 8, Family Planning,** features 14 lists, such as "Reasons Why Teens Choose Abstinence" (152), "Advantages and Disadvantages of Contraceptive Methods" (157), "Who Should Not Use Oral Contraceptives" (162), and "Risk of Death Associated With Birth Control Methods, Pregnancy, and Abortion" (163).

➡ **Section 9, Pregnancy and Childbirth,** provides 22 lists, including "Fetal Development Stages" (166), "Special Food Needs During Pregnancy" (171), "Leading Categories of Birth Defects" (178), and "Teen Pregnancy Statistics" (183).

➡ **Section 10, Relationships and Communication,** includes 17 lists on topics dealing with family relationships, friendship, marriage, and methods of communication. Some of the lists are "Barriers to Good Communication" (188), "Refusal Skills" (190), "Relationship Skills" (192), and "Signs of Troubled Relationships" (196).

➡ **Section 11, Stress Management and Self-Esteem,** provides 24 lists, such as "Adolescent Life-Change-Event Scale" (204), "Factors Influencing Stress" (205), "Time-Management Techniques for Students" (212), and "Healthful Ways to Deal With Emotions" (222).

➡ **Section 12, Violence Prevention,** offers 18 lists, including "Reasons for Teen Violence" (227), "Facts About Rape" (235), "Symptoms of Domestic Abuse" (238), and "Public Health Service Agencies and Sources of Information" (244).

➡ **Section 13, Substance Abuse,** includes 27 lists dealing with alcohol and other drugs, tobacco, and decision making. Examples are "Factors That Discourage Drug Use" (245), "Sources of Steroids and Reasons for Their Use" (253), "Methods and Programs to Quit Smoking" (266), and "Common Drug Treatment Approaches" (268).

➡ **Section 14, Aging, Death, Dying, and Suicide,** offers 20 lists, such as "Leading Causes of Death" (278), "Stages in the Acceptance of Death" (281), "Ways to Help Others Grieve" (284), and "Warning Signs of Suicide" (288).

We hope you'll find these collected lists from our years of experience in teaching health to be useful in your daily planning and instruction.

Patricia Rizzo-Toner
Marian D. Milliken

CONTENTS

SECTION 1
SYSTEMS OF THE BODY

SECTION 2
HUMAN SEXUALITY

SECTION 3
DIET AND NUTRITION

SECTION 4
CONSUMER HEALTH

SECTION 5

FIRST AID AND SAFETY

SECTION 6
DISEASES AND DISORDERS

SECTION 7
SEXUALLY TRANSMITTED INFECTIONS, HIV, AND AIDS

SECTION 8

FAMILY PLANNING

SECTION 9
PREGNANCY AND CHILDBIRTH

SECTION 10
RELATIONSHIPS AND COMMUNICATION

SECTION 11
STRESS MANAGEMENT AND SELF-ESTEEM

SECTION 12

VIOLENCE PREVENTION

SECTION 13

SUBSTANCE ABUSE

SECTION 14
AGING, DEATH, DYING, AND SUICIDE

Section 1

SYSTEMS OF THE BODY

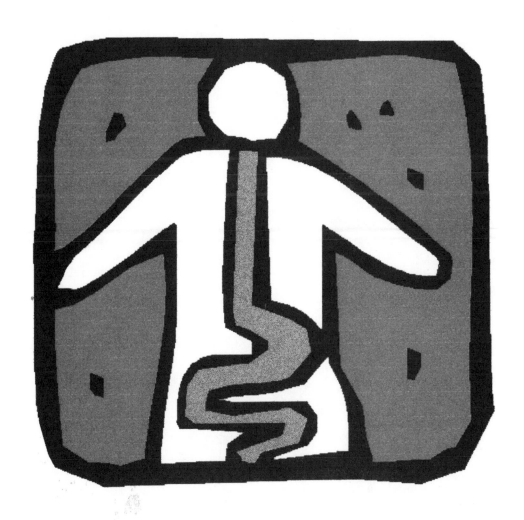

1. SYSTEMS OF THE BODY

Skeletal System
Muscular System
Nervous System
Endocrine System
Circulatory System
Lymphatic System
Respiratory System
Digestive System
Urinary System
Reproductive System

2. TYPES OF BODY TISSUE

EPITHELIAL TISSUE   Groups of cells that cover parts of the body.

CONNECTIVE TISSUE   Groups of cells that support the body and connect one part of the body to another.

MUSCLE TISSUE   Groups of muscle cells that work together to cause movement.

NERVOUS TISSUE   Groups of nerve cells that carry messages throughout the body and also receive impressions from the environment.

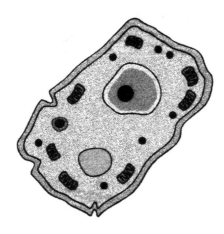

3. FUNCTIONS AND STRUCTURE OF THE SKIN

FUNCTIONS OF THE SKIN

➡ Serves as a waterproof covering
➡ Protects internal organs
➡ Protects internal tissues
➡ Protects body from invading pathogens
➡ Provides protection against ultraviolet rays of the sun
➡ Regulates body temperature
➡ Serves as a major sense organ

STRUCTURE OF THE SKIN

EPIDERMIS	Outer, thinner layer of skin, made up of both dead and living cells.
DERMIS	Inner, thicker layer of skin.
HYPODERMIS	Attaches skin to bone and muscle.

4. FUNCTIONS AND STRUCTURE OF THE SKELETAL SYSTEM

FUNCTIONS OF THE SKELETAL SYSTEM

➡ Allows movement
➡ Provides a supporting framework
➡ Protects delicate internal organs
➡ Provides storage for essential body minerals
➡ Red and white blood cells produced in the red marrow

STRUCTURE OF THE SKELETAL SYSTEM

AXIAL SKELETON	Includes the bones of the skull, the sternum, the ribs, and the vertebrae.
APPENDICULAR SKELETON	Includes the 126 bones of the shoulders, arms, hands, hips, legs, and feet.
CARTILAGE	A strong, flexible material that provides a smooth surface at the joint.
PERIOSTEUM	A tough membrane that adheres to the outer surface of bone, provides nourishment, and produces bone cells.
LIGAMENTS	Strong bands or cords of tissue that connect the bones at a movable joint.
TENDONS	Bands of fiber that connect muscles to bones.

5. TYPES OF BONES AND JOINTS

TYPES OF BONES

LONG BONES   Strong bones, such as the femur, found in the arms and legs.

SHORT BONES   Over half of which can be found in the hands and feet, are as broad as they are long.

FLAT BONES   Thin, flat bones, such as the ribs and skull, which serve to protect vital body organs.

IRREGULAR BONES   Have shapes that do not fit with the other types of bones, such as vertebrae.

TYPES OF JOINTS

IMMOVABLE JOINTS   Such as the joints in the skull, do not move.

SLIGHTLY MOVABLE JOINTS   Such as the joints in the vertebrae, allow for a small amount of movement.

BALL-AND-SOCKET JOINTS   Such as the hip or shoulder joint, which allow limited movement in any direction.

PIVOT JOINTS   Allow the head to turn on the spine, for example; one bone rotates around another.

GLIDING JOINTS   Such as in the hand and foot, allow bones to slide over one another.

HINGE JOINTS   Such as the knee joint, which allow movement in only one plane.

6. MAJOR BONES OF THE BODY

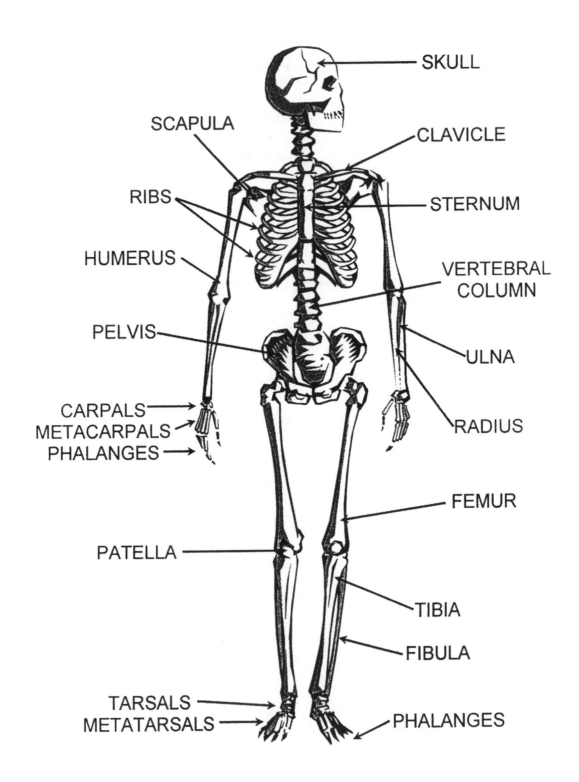

SKULL

SCAPULA

CLAVICLE

RIBS

STERNUM

HUMERUS

VERTEBRAL
COLUMN

PELVIS

ULNA

CARPALS
METACARPALS
PHALANGES

RADIUS

FEMUR

PATELLA

TIBIA

FIBULA

TARSALS
METATARSALS

PHALANGES

7. MAJOR SKELETAL MUSCLES, MUSCLE TYPES, AND THEIR FUNCTIONS

MUSCLE TYPES AND THEIR FUNCTIONS

SMOOTH MUSCLES (UNSTRIATED MUSCLES)   Involuntary muscles such as in the blood vessels and intestines.

CARDIAC MUSCLE   Involuntary type of striated tissue that forms the walls of the heart.

SKELETAL MUSCLES   Voluntary muscles attached to bones; cause body movement.

FLEXOR   Muscle that bends a limb at a joint.

EXTENSOR   Muscle that straightens a limb at a joint.

MAJOR SKELETAL MUSCLES

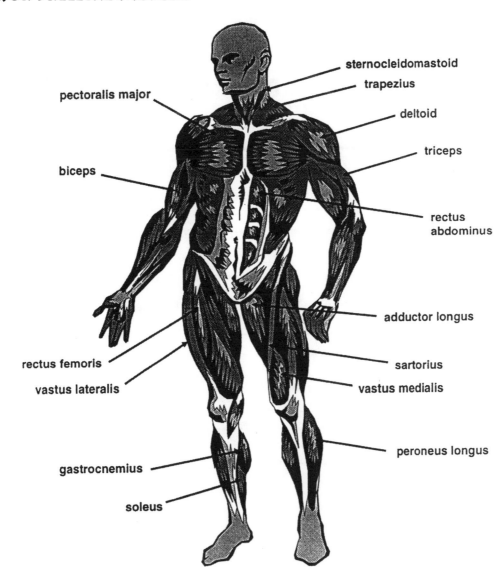

8. FUNCTIONS AND STRUCTURE OF THE NERVOUS SYSTEM

FUNCTIONS OF THE NERVOUS SYSTEM

➠ Body's communication and control center

➠ Transmits information by nerve impulses from one nerve cell to another throughout the body

➠ Senses changes inside and outside the body in order for the body to adjust quickly to internal or external changes

STRUCTURE OF THE NERVOUS SYSTEM

➠ Central Nervous System (CNS) includes the brain and spinal cord

➠ Peripheral Nervous System (PNS) consists of nerves and ganglia (groups of nerve cell bodies)

9. FUNCTIONS AND STRUCTURES OF THE NEURONS

FUNCTIONS OF THE NEURONS

SENSORY NEURONS	Receive stimuli, such as sounds, and send impulses to the spinal cord and brain. Sensory receptors for heat, cold, pain, hearing, taste, sight, smell, touch, and balance.
INTERNEURONS	Relay impulses from sensory neurons to motor neurons.
MOTOR NEURONS	Carry impulses from interneurons to muscles and glands.

STRUCTURE OF THE NEURONS

CELL BODY	Has a nucleus and is the center for receiving and sending nerve impulses.
DENDRITE	Receives and carries impulses toward the cell body.
AXON	Carries impulses away from the cell body.

10. MAIN DIVISIONS OF THE BRAIN

CEREBRUM

The upper and main part of the brain; controls muscular activity and receives sensory input.

FOUR LOBES OF CEREBRUM:

Frontal—controls voluntary movements, motivation, mood, and aggression.

Parietal—controls sensory information and kinesthetic sense.

Occipital—controls vision.

Temporal—controls sense of smell, hearing, memory, thought, and judgment.

CEREBELLUM

The lower rear part of the brain; coordinates movement and helps the body maintain its balance.

BRAIN STEM

Connects the spinal cord to the brain; includes the medulla oblongata, pons, midbrain, and interbrain.

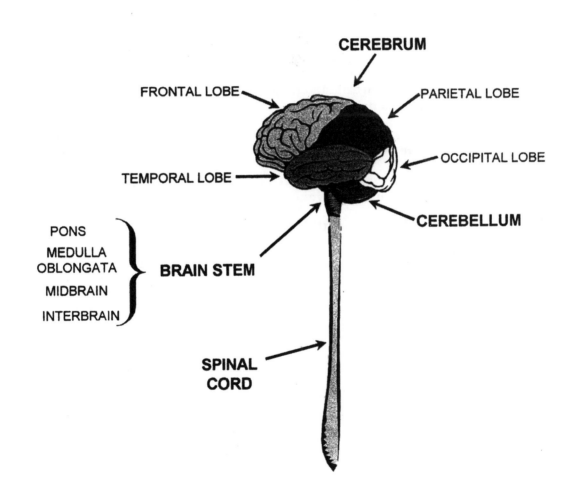

11. FUNCTIONS AND MAJOR GLANDS OF THE ENDOCRINE SYSTEM

FUNCTIONS OF THE ENDOCRINE SYSTEM

➡ Regulates body functions through the use of glands

➡ Secretes substances into ducts to be carried to specific areas of the body

➡ Secretes hormones that regulate activities of various body cells

MAJOR GLANDS OF THE ENDOCRINE SYSTEM

PITUITARY GLAND   A pea-sized gland located at the base of the brain that regulates activities of other endocrine glands and controls body growth.

THYROID GLAND   An H-shaped gland in the front of the neck that secretes a hormone that controls the speed at which body cells work.

PARATHYROID GLANDS   Four small glands located behind the thyroid gland that regulate the calcium content of the blood.

ADRENAL GLANDS   Glands located on the kidneys that regulate the use of carbohydrates and salt, and prepare the body for emergencies by producing adrenaline.

PANCREAS   A digestive gland that secretes pancreatic juice into the intestine and insulin into the bloodstream.

OVARIES   Female sex glands that produce ova and the female hormones estrogen and progesterone.

TESTES   Male sex glands that produce sperm and the male hormone testosterone.

12. FUNCTIONS AND STRUCTURE OF THE CARDIOVASCULAR SYSTEM

FUNCTIONS OF THE CARDIOVASCULAR SYSTEM

➡ Heart pumps blood to all body cells through the circulatory system

➡ Blood vessels carry oxygen and nutrients from the lungs and small intestines to all body cells

➡ Carbon dioxide and other waste products are carried away from the body cells to the lungs and the kidneys, where they are released from the body

STRUCTURE OF THE CARDIOVASCULAR SYSTEM

HEART	Fist-sized muscular organ that is enclosed in a loose-fitting sac called the pericardium.
BLOOD	Fluid that delivers oxygen, hormones, and nutrients to the cells and carries away the wastes that the cells produce.
BLOOD VESSELS	80,000-mile-long system through which blood is distributed to the body.
ARTERIES	Largest blood vessels, which carry blood away from the heart.
CAPILLARIES	Smallest blood vessels, which link arteries and veins.
VEINS	Blood vessels that carry blood back to the heart.

© 1999 by The Center for Applied Research in Education

13. PATH OF BLOOD THROUGH THE HEART

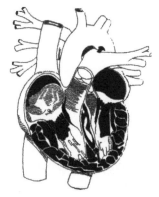

PULMONARY CIRCULATION
Flow of blood from the heart to lungs and back to the heart.
Inferior and superior vena cava return blood containing waste products from the body cells to right atrium.
Right atrium fills and contracts.
Blood flows into right ventricle.
Ventricle pumps blood to lungs through pulmonary arteries.
Carbon dioxide and oxygen are exchanged in the lungs.
Oxygen-rich blood returns to the left atrium in the pulmonary veins.

SYSTEM CIRCULATION
Moves blood to all body tissues.
Oxygen-rich blood flows from the left atrium to the left ventricle.
Left ventricle pumps blood through the aorta to all parts of the body.

14. STRUCTURE OF THE BLOOD AND BLOOD TYPES

Structure of the Blood

PLASMA	Largest, and fluid, portion of the blood, in which the red blood cells, white blood cells, and platelets are suspended.
RED BLOOD CELLS	Carry oxygen from the lungs to all of the body cells.
WHITE BLOOD CELLS	Produced in the red bone marrow, destroy invading pathogens.
PLATELETS	Smallest parts of the blood, produce small fibers, called fibrin, that assist in clot formation to prevent blood loss.

Blood Types

TYPE A	
TYPE B	
TYPE AB	Universal recipient, able to receive any blood type.
TYPE O	Universal donor, donate blood to any blood type.

15. FUNCTIONS AND STRUCTURE OF THE LYMPHATIC SYSTEM

Functions of the Lymphatic System

- Maintains the body's fluid balance by carrying excess fluid away from body tissues
- Assists the body in its defense against pathogens

Structure of the Lymphatic System

LYMPHATIC VESSELS	Carry lymph to lymph ducts in neck and chest.
LYMPH NODES	Masses of tissue which serve to filter lymph before it returns to the blood.
LYMPH	Clear yellow fluid that fills the areas around the cells.
LYMPHOCYTES	White blood cells that serve to destroy invading pathogens.
T-CELLS	Produced in bone marrow, transported to thymus, release a toxin that weakens the pathogen.
B-CELLS	Produce antibodies that destroy or neutralize invading pathogens.
SPLEEN	Organ that keeps the body free of foreign substances and stores B-cells.
TONSILS	Mass of lymphatic tissue that filters out pathogens that enter the mouth and nose.
THYMUS GLAND	Produces lymphocytes in infants and children.

16. FUNCTIONS AND STRUCTURE OF THE RESPIRATORY SYSTEM

FUNCTIONS OF THE RESPIRATORY SYSTEM

➡ Exchanges oxygen and carbon dioxide between the air in the lungs and the blood
➡ Exchanges oxygen and carbon dioxide between the blood and the body cells

STRUCTURE OF THE RESPIRATORY SYSTEM

NASAL CAVITY	The inner area of the nasal passage where air is warmed and cleaned by cilia and mucous membranes.
PHARYNX	The upper part of the throat between the mouth and the esophagus.
LARYNX	The voice box, which lies in the front of the throat and is seen on the outside as the Adam's apple.
TRACHEA	The main tube through which air passes to and from the lungs, also called the windpipe.
BRONCHI	Bronchial tubes that lead to the lungs.
LUNGS	Organs that contain bronchial tubes, bronchioles, and aveoli in which exchange of oxygen and carbon dioxide takes place.
DIAPHRAGM	Muscle that separates the chest and abdominal cavities.

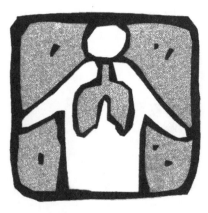

14

17. FUNCTIONS AND STRUCTURE OF THE DIGESTIVE SYSTEM

FUNCTIONS OF THE DIGESTIVE SYSTEM

➡ Physically and chemically breaks down food into smaller pieces

➡ Moves digested food from the digestive tract into the circulatory system through the process of absorption

➡ Eliminates undigested food and waste products from the body

STRUCTURE OF THE DIGESTIVE SYSTEM

MOUTH	Contains teeth, which break food into smaller pieces by chewing (mastication), which allows food to be swallowed.
SALIVARY GLANDS	Secrete saliva, which begins the breakdown of carbohydrates and helps food to move down the throat.
TONGUE	Muscular organ that prepares food to be swallowed and contains the taste buds (sweet, sour, salty, and bitter).
ESOPHAGUS	Tube through which food passes in going from the pharnyx to the stomach.
STOMACH	Muscular pouch in which food is stored and mixed with gastric juices to form chyme.
SMALL INTESTINE	Long tube extending from the stomach to the colon, which is the main site for the absorption of food.
LARGE INTESTINE	Tube located below the small intestine that removes water from undigested food and eliminates waste from the body.

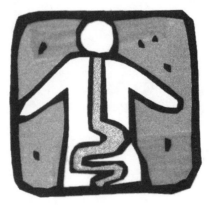

18. FUNCTIONS AND STRUCTURE OF THE URINARY SYSTEM

FUNCTIONS OF THE URINARY SYSTEM

➡ Filters wastes from the circulatory system

➡ Eliminates wastes from the body in the form of urine

STRUCTURE OF THE URINARY SYSTEM

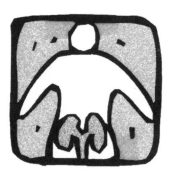

KIDNEYS	Two organs located on either side of the spine in the small of the back; filter impurities from the blood and produce urine.
URETERS	Two long tubes that carry liquid wastes from the kidneys to the bladder.
BLADDER	Sac that collects urine from the kidney in preparation for excretion.
URETHRA	Tube that carries urine from the bladder to the outside of the body.

19. FUNCTIONS AND STRUCTURE OF THE TEETH

FUNCTIONS OF THE TEETH

➡ Form the shape and structure of the mouth

➡ Begin the process of digestion by breaking food down into smaller pieces through the process of chewing (mastication)

STRUCTURE OF THE TEETH

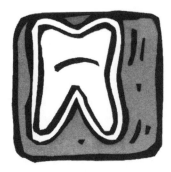

PERIODONTIUM	Area immediately around the teeth; includes gums, periodontal ligament, and jaw bone.
CROWN	Visible part of the tooth, covered by enamel.
ROOT	Tooth section including pulp cavity containing nerves and blood vessels.

20. STRUCTURE OF THE EYE

SCLERA   White outer membrane of the eye that helps the eye to keep its shape.

CORNEA   Exposed and transparent portion of the eye, which contains nerve endings.

CHOROID   Layer of tissue in the eye that contains blood vessels.

IRIS   Colored ring containing two sets of muscles that control the size of the pupil and the amount of light admitted through it.

SUSPENSORY LIGAMENTS   Ligaments located behind the pupil that serve to hold the lens.

CILIARY MUSCLES   Control the shape of the lens.

AQUEOUS HUMOR   Watery fluid that fills the cavity between the cornea and the lens.

VITREOUS HUMOR   Fluid located behind the lens that keeps the eyeball firm.

RETINA   Light-sensitive tissue at the back of the eye.

OPTIC NERVE   Nerve located at the back of the eye; transmits visual images to the brain.

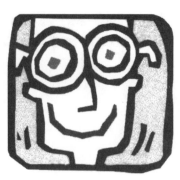

21. STRUCTURE OF THE EAR

OUTER EAR

AURICLE

Fleshy outer area of the ear.

EXTERNAL AUDITORY CANAL

Passageway leading to the eardrum, containing fine hairs and wax-producing glands that filter out foreign substances.

MIDDLE EAR

OSSICLES

Three small bones connecting the eardrum to the inner ear.

MALLEUS

Connected to the eardrum, the largest of the ossicles.

INCUS

Connects the malleus to the innermost bone, the stapes.

STAPES

Stirrup-shaped bone attached to the inner ear; the smallest bone in the body.

MASTOID PROCESS

Small spaces in the bones behind the middle ear that connect with the inner ear.

EUSTACHIAN TUBE

Connects the nasal cavity in the back of the throat with the middle ear.

INNER EAR

VESTIBULE

Contains the semicircular canals and controls balance.

SEMICIRCULAR CANALS

Three structures containing nerve fibers that transmit information to the brain.

COCHLEA

Spiral-shaped structure that contains hearing receptors.

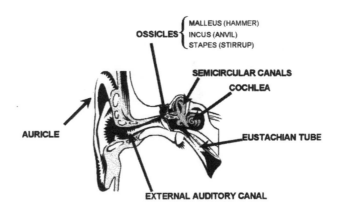

22. PATH OF SOUND WAVES THROUGH THE EAR

➡ Sound waves enter the external auditory canal through the auricle

➡ Sound waves cause the eardrum to vibrate

➡ Vibrations are carried across the middle ear by the malleus, incus, and stapes to the opening between the middle and inner ear (the oval window)

➡ Sound vibrations cause the stapes to move in and out of the oval window, causing fluid in the cochlea to move

➡ Tiny fibers within the cochlea are set into motion by the sound waves

➡ Fibers cause a vibration in the hearing receptors, which stimulates the nerves attached to them

➡ The nerves send messages through the auditory nerve to the temporal lobe

➡ Sounds are interpreted in the temporal lobe of the brain

23. BODY SENSES

SIGHT   The ability to perceive images by means of the eye.

HEARING   The ability to perceive sound by means of the ear.

TOUCH   The ability to feel through contact with the skin.

SMELL   The ability to perceive scents by means of the olfactory nerves.

TASTE   The ability to savor flavors by means of the taste buds.

24. BODY PARTS COMPARED TO AUTOMOBILE PARTS

As noted by Mitchell Wilson in *The Human Body*, many of the parts of the body perform the same functions that the parts of an automobile perform, as shown below.

Rotary joints	=	Wheels
Muscles	=	Cylinders
Nerve endings	=	Spark plugs
Arteries	=	Fuel line
Lungs	=	Carburetor
Heart	=	Fuel pump
Digestive system	=	Fuel system
Nerve impulses	=	Ignition
Waste	=	Exhaust
Oxygen	=	Air intake

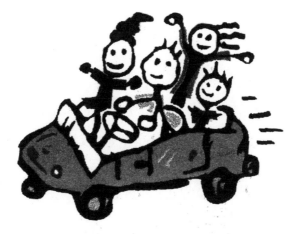

25. INTERESTING FACTS ABOUT THE HUMAN BODY

➡ The heart beats over 100,000 times each day and pumps about 2,000 gallons of blood each day.

➡ The average resting pulse of females is 2 to 15 beats per minute faster than the average resting pulse of males.

➡ The better the body conditioning, the lower the pulse; athletes may have a resting pulse of 45 beats per minute.

➡ The largest blood vessel in the body, the aorta, measures about one inch in diameter.

➡ Woman have fewer total red blood cells and about 15% less hemoglobin than men.

➡ Skeletal muscles account for about 40% of a man's body weight and about 23% for a woman.

➡ Testosterone, the male hormone, is responsible for muscle bulkiness in men; women also have testosterone, but about 1/10th that of men.

➡ Men and woman have the same number of ribs—24.

➡ Babies have 350 bones at birth, but many join during growth and at adulthood, they have 206. If you count the 6 ossicles (little bones), 3 in each ear, the total is 212.

➡ The digestive process can go on without a stomach because most food is digested in the small intestine.

➡ The stomach's hydrochloric acid can dissolve materials as strong as steel.

➡ The stomach of an average-sized person has a capacity for about one quart of food.

➡ In the rapid growth period of adolescence, the feet and hands have a growth spurt before legs and arms lengthen.

➡ Also during adolescent growth, the nose reaches its adult length before the jaw begins to thicken.

➡ The average human being sheds about 1 1/2 pounds of skin particles in a year.

➡ Nerves link more than 600 muscles to the brain and spinal cord.

➡ Nerve impulses move along the nerve fibers as fast as 115 feet per second.

➡ The liver detoxifies 1/2 ounce of pure alcohol per hour; taking another liquid or food will not help a person become sober more quickly.

➡ The Greek physician Galen (about 129 AD–210 AD) was the first to discover that arteries carry blood and not air. (For over 400 years, the Alexandrian school of medicine had taught that the arteries are full of air.)

➡ Galen was appointed physician to the school of gladiators around the year 157 AD, which some say made him the first sports medicine specialist.

SECTION 2

HUMAN SEXUALITY

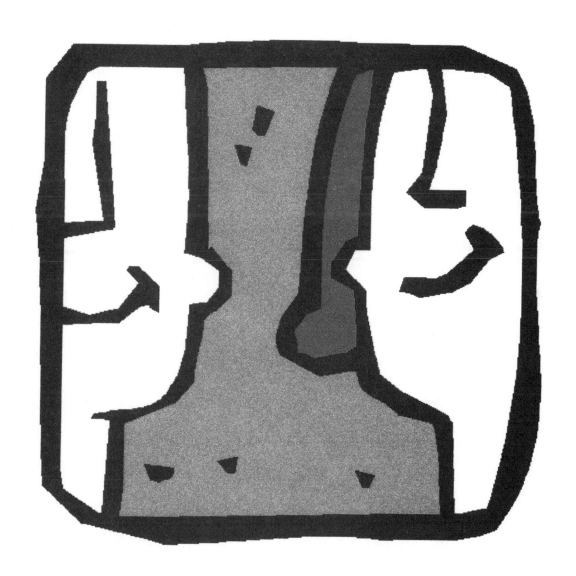

26. ORGANS OF THE MALE REPRODUCTIVE SYSTEM

ORGAN	FUNCTION
SCROTUM	Sac that holds the testes and regulates the temperature of the testes.
TESTES	Two structures inside the scrotum that secrete testosterone and produce sperm.
SEMINIFEROUS TUBULES	Tubes inside the testes that contain and convey sperm.
EPIDIDYMIS	Structure on the upper surface of each testicle that stores sperm.
VAS DEFERENS	Two tubes that serve as a passageway for sperm and storage of sperm.
SEMINAL VESICLES	Two small glands that secrete a sugary fluid rich in fructose that provides energy for sperm.
EJACULATORY DUCT	Short tube that passes into the prostate gland and opens into the urethra.
PROSTATE GLAND	Gland that produces an alkaline fluid that helps sperm to live longer.
COWPER'S GLANDS (BULBOURETHRAL GLANDS)	Two small glands on each side of the urethra that secrete a lubricating fluid.
URETHRA	Tube from the bladder to the tip of the penis that serves as a passageway for both semen and urine.
PENIS	The male organ of intercourse.

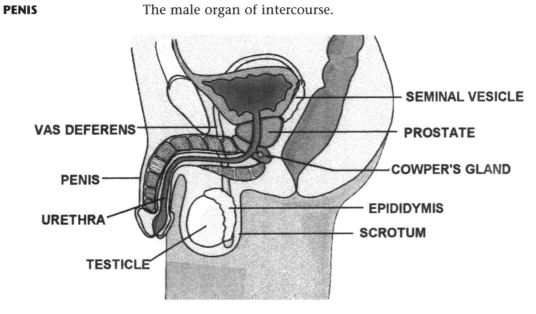

27. COMPONENTS OF SEMEN

➡ Sperm cells
➡ Nutrient fluid from the seminal vesicle
➡ Acidic fluid from the prostate gland
➡ Lubricating and neutralizing fluid from the Cowper's glands

28. PATH OF SPERM CELLS

➡ Produced in the testes
➡ Stored in the epididymis
➡ Travel through the vas deferens
➡ Combine with fluid from the seminal vesicle
➡ Combine with fluid from the prostate gland
➡ Combine with fluid from the Cowper's glands
➡ Now called semen, travels through the urethra in the penis
➡ Leaves the body through the opening in the penis during ejaculation

29. MALE CHANGES DURING PUBERTY

Puberty is the stage of growth and development in which males and females become capable of producing children. In males, testosterone, the male hormone is released into the bloodstream from the testes and causes the following male secondary sex characteristics to develop during puberty:

➡ Larger muscles
➡ Longer, heavier bones
➡ Thicker, tougher skin
➡ Deeper voice
➡ Growth of body hair
➡ Development of pubic hair
➡ Greater muscle mass
➡ V-shaped torso
➡ Enlargement of penis, scrotum, and testes
➡ Increased metabolic rate
➡ Sex drive
➡ Ejaculation of semen

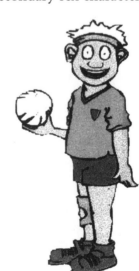

© 1999 by The Center for Applied Research in Education

30. MALE PHYSIOLOGY

The male reproductive organs produce a hormone called testosterone, produce sperm cells, and transport the sperm to the female. Male physiology involves erection, orgasm, and ejaculation.

ERECTION   An involuntary process that occurs when the spongy tissue inside the male penis becomes engorged, causing the penis to become stiff and hard.

ORGASM   An explosive discharge at the peak of sexual excitement that is marked by rhythmic contractions and a sense of release. This usually occurs with ejaculation.

EJACULATION   The sudden expulsion of semen from the male penis.

31. PROBLEMS OF THE MALE REPRODUCTIVE SYSTEM

INGUINAL HERNIA   A common hernia of the male reproductive system that occurs when the intestines rupture through a weak spot in the abdominal wall and push into the scrotum.

ENLARGED PROSTATE GLAND   A condition, occurring as a result of a tumor, infection, or old age, that causes the prostate gland to increase in size. This condition causes difficulty in urination as the enlarged gland begins to squeeze the urethra.

CANCER OF THE PROSTATE GLAND   An uncontrolled growth of cells in the prostate gland. This is often a site of cancer in older males.

TESTICULAR CANCER   An uncontrolled growth of cells in the testes. This occurs most frequently in males between the ages of 15 and 34.

ANDROPAUSE   The decrease in male sexual function due to diminished testosterone levels.

STERILITY   The inability to reproduce due to poor-quality sperm, or too few sperm.

CRYPTORCHIDISM   A condition in which the testes do not descend into the scrotum before birth. Treatment is available to prevent sterility.

32. SOME CAUSES OF MALE STERILITY

A sterile male can function sexually but cannot reproduce.

➡ Extreme temperature changes
➡ Low sperm production
➡ Exposure to certain chemicals
➡ Contracting mumps as an adult
➡ Smoking
➡ Sexually transmitted infection complications
➡ Malformation of the epididymis, vas deferens, Cowper's glands, or prostate gland
➡ Undescended testes

33. SIGNS OF PROSTATE AND TESTICULAR CANCER

PROSTATE CANCER

Usually none at first

Loss in force of urine

Dribbling

Increased frequency of urination

Blood in urine

Passing urine at night

Pain in the pelvic area

Lower back pain

TESTICULAR CANCER

Enlargement of one teste

Presence of pain

Dull ache in lower abdomen and groin

Hard lumps or nodules on testes

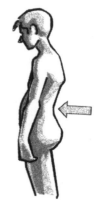

34. MALE SEXUAL CONCERNS

IMPOTENCE The inability to maintain an erection in order to have intercourse. This condition can be due to stress, illness, or exhaustion.

NOCTURNAL EMISSIONS Spontaneous ejaculations that occur during sleep. Also called "wet dreams."

PENIS SIZE Some males worry unnecessarily about the size of the penis. Penis size has nothing to do with adequate sexual function.

ANABOLIC STEROIDS The use of anabolic steroids (drugs produced from male sex hormones) can cause atrophy of the testicles, as well as, liver damage and kidney failure.

CIRCUMCISION The surgical removal of the foreskin from the penis. Uncircumcised males have a greater chance of having some infections.

SMEGMA A cheesy substance that forms under the foreskin. If smegma is not controlled by regular washing, it develops an odor.

Microorganisms that cause infection may collect in smegma.

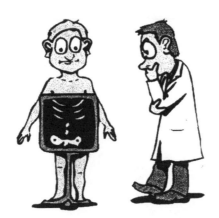

35. THE EXTERNAL ORGANS OF THE FEMALE REPRODUCTIVE SYSTEM

ORGAN	FUNCTION
VULVA	The external female reproductive organs.
MONS PUBIS	Soft tissue that covers the pubic bone and serves as a protective cushion for the reproductive organs.
LABIA MAJORA	The outer folds of skin that surround the opening of the vagina.
LABIA MINORA	The inner folds of skin that surround the opening of the vagina.
CLITORIS	A small, highly sensitive organ located between the labia minora, or inner folds.
URETHRAL OPENING	The opening at the end of the urethra. The urethra is a tube that carries urine from the bladder to the outside of the body.
HYMEN	A thin membrane that stretches across the vaginal opening.
BREASTS	Organs composed of fatty tissue that are sensitive and that provide milk for a newborn baby.
BREASTS	Organs composed of fatty tissue that are sensitive and that provide milk for a newborn baby.
BARTHOLIN'S GLANDS	A pair of glands located near the labia minora which secrete fluid during sexual excitement.

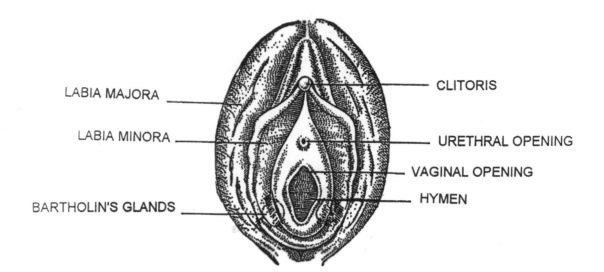

36. THE INTERNAL ORGANS OF THE FEMALE REPRODUCTIVE SYSTEM

VAGINA A muscular, elastic tube approximately 3–4 inches long that extends from the uterus to the outside of the body. The vagina serves as a passageway for male sperm, the birth canal, and the female organ of intercourse.

UTERUS A hollow, muscular, pear-shaped organ that prepares each month to receive a fertilized egg, houses the fetus during pregnancy, and pushes the baby out during childbirth.

CERVIX The lower portion of the uterus that is a common site of cancer in females.

FALLOPIAN TUBES Two muscular tubes through which the egg cell moves from the ovary to the uterus.

ENDOMETRIUM The inside lining of the uterus.

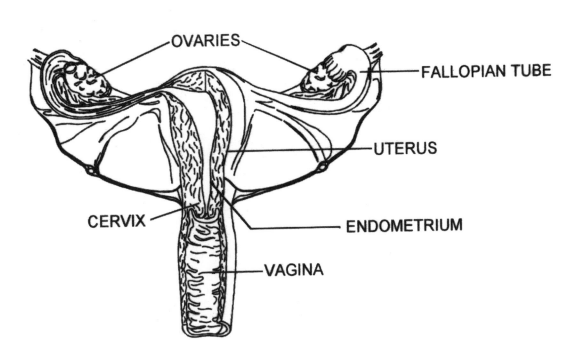

37. FEMALE CHANGES DURING PUBERTY

Puberty is the stage of growth and development in which males and females become capable of producing children. In females, estrogen, the female hormone is released into the bloodstream from the ovaries and causes the following female secondary sex characteristics to develop during puberty:

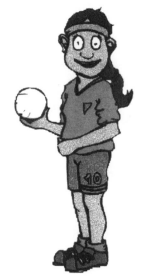

⇒ Breasts
⇒ Broadening of pelvis
⇒ Soft and smooth skin
⇒ Deposition of fat in the thighs and buttocks
⇒ Pubic hair
⇒ Sex drive
⇒ Ovulation
⇒ Menstruation

38. FEMALE PHYSIOLOGY

The female reproductive organs produce egg cells (ova) and secrete the hormones estrogen and progesterone. Female physiology involves ovulation, menstruation, fertilization, pregnancy, and childbirth.

OVULATION	The release of a mature egg cell (ovum) from the ovary that usually occurs once each month.
MENSTRUATION	The process by which the uterus sheds its lining. The cycle consists of the lining of the uterus thickening in preparation for the possibility of a fertilized egg, followed by ovulation. If the egg is not fertilized, the lining of the uterus begins to break down, and eventually blood and tissue leave the body. The cycle lasts approximately 28 days.
FERTILIZATION	The union of an egg and a sperm cell that occurs in the Fallopian tube. This process is also called conception.
PREGNANCY	The process by which a fertilized egg grows and develops in the mother's uterus and forms a new individual. In humans, this process lasts about nine months.
CHILDBIRTH	The delivery of the baby from the mother's uterus.

39. PROBLEMS OF THE FEMALE REPRODUCTIVE SYSTEM

AMENORRHEA   The absence of menstruation.

DYSMENORRHEA   Extremely painful menstruation.

MENORRHAGIA   An abnormally heavy menstrual flow.

PREMENSTRUAL SYNDROME (PMS)   A combination of severe physical and emotional symptoms occurring on the days before and during menstruation; common symptoms include

Bloating	Swelling of breasts	Fatigue
Weight gain	Constipation	Lack of concentration
Headaches	Edema	
Cravings for food	Anxiety	Depression

TOXIC SHOCK SYNDROME (TSS)   A severe, possibly life-threatening combination of physical and psychological symptoms occurring on the days before and during menstruation. This condition is also due to certain types of tampons or failure to change tampons for an extended period of time.

MASTODYNIA   The painful swelling and tenderness of the breasts during the menstrual cycle.

CYST   A sac that forms when fluid becomes trapped in a lymph duct.

FIBROADENOMA   A lump that forms when fluid becomes trapped in a lymph duct.

BREAST CANCER   A disease in which malignant tumors grow in the breast tissue.

UTERINE CANCER   A disease in which malignant tumors grow on or in the uterus.

CERVICAL CANCER   A disease in which malignant tumors grow on or in the cervix, which is the lower part of the uterus.

OVARIAN CANCER   A disease in which there are cancerous cells and tumors in one or both ovaries.

VAGINAL CANCER   A disease in which there are cancerous cells and tumors present in the vagina.

VAGINITIS   An irritation or inflammation of the vagina.

CYSTITIS   Inflammation of the urinary bladder.

ENDOMETRIOSIS   A condition in which the endometrial tissue is abnormally present outside the uterus.

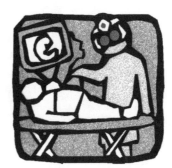

FIBROIDS   Slow-growing, noncancerous (benign) growths in the uterus.

40. RISK FACTORS FOR BREAST CANCER

➡ Being older than 50

➡ Having a family history of breast cancer

➡ Starting menstruation before age 12

➡ Having no pregnancies

➡ Having a first child born after the age of 30

➡ Beginning menopause after age 50

➡ Being obese

➡ Having a high percentage of body fat

➡ Having a high-fat diet

➡ Having cancer in one breast

Source: National Cancer Institute.

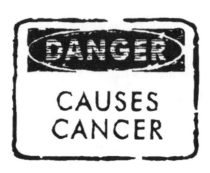

41. FEMALE SEXUAL CONCERNS

BREAST SIZE   Some females worry unnecessarily about the size of their breasts. Breast size has nothing to do with sexual function. The amount of fat tissue in the breasts is responsible for the variation in breast size.

VIRGINITY   The absence of the hymen is not a sign that a female is no longer a virgin. The hymen usually tears during first intercourse, but may be torn or absent, in some women, prior to first intercourse.

MENOPAUSE   The cessation of the monthly menstrual cycle that occurs sometime after a woman reaches age 45–50. The ovaries stop producing egg cells, the hormone level decreases, and eventually menstruation stops.

42. SYMPTOMS OF MENOPAUSE

HOT FLASHES A warm and sweaty feeling that occurs when the arteries dilate and blood rushes to the skin surface.

VAGINAL DRYNESS A loss of elasticity in the vaginal walls causes the mucous membranes in the vagina to thin out. This may cause discomfort or pain during intercourse.

INFECTION Due to a lower production of estrogen, the vagina is more susceptible to infection.

OTHER SYMPTOMS: Inability to sleep

Fatigue	Anxiety
Headaches	Depression
Numbness in the hands and feet	Itching or burning skin
	Short-term memory loss

43. TYPES OF EXAMINATIONS AND PROCEDURES

BIOPSY Removal of tissue from a lump to determine if cancer cells are present.

BIMANUAL PELVIC EXAMINATION A physician inserts the index and middle finger of one hand into the vagina and palpates the abdomen with the other hand. This is done to check reproductive organs.

BLOOD PRESSURE CHECK A procedure to determine how much force the blood is exerting against the walls of the arteries.

BLOOD TESTS A blood sample is taken and sent to a laboratory to determine the hemoglobin level, the Rh factor, and/or the level of triglycerides and cholesterol in the bloodstream.

BREAST EXAMINATION An exam in which a physician checks the breasts for growths, lumps, or discharge.

BREAST SELF-EXAMINATION An exam in which a female visually checks her breasts, palpates them to detect any growths or lumps, and squeezes her nipples to check for a clear or bloody discharge.

CASTRATION The removal of the testes.

CERVICAL BIOPSY The surgical removal of tissue from the cervix for examination.

CIRCUMCISION The surgical removal of the foreskin of the penis.

COLPOSCOPY An exam in which a microscope is used to detect the presence of abnormal or cancerous cells.

CRYOSURGERY Tissue from the cervix is frozen and cancerous cells are removed.

DIGITAL RECTAL EXAMINATION	An exam in which the doctor inserts a finger into the rectum of a male to examine the condition of the prostate and rectum for signs of cancer.
DILATATION AND CURETTAGE (D & C)	A surgical procedure in which the opening of the cervix is dilated and a metal loop curette is inserted to scrape away the uterine lining.
HEALTH HISTORY	A detailed description of a person's health status.
HYSTERECTOMY	The surgical removal of the uterus.
LUMPECTOMY	The surgical removal of a lump and a small amount of the surrounding tissue of the breast.
MAMMOGRAPHY	A highly sensitive X-ray used to detect breast lumps.
MASTECTOMY	The surgical removal of the breast.
NEEDLE ASPIRATION	A needle is inserted into a breast lump to determine if fluid is detected. If fluid is detected, the lump or cyst is drained.
OPHORECTOMY	The surgical removal of one or both ovaries.
ORCHIECTOMY	The operation in which one or both testes are removed.
PAP SMEAR	A test to detect cervical cancer, in which cells are scraped from the cervix and examined.
PELVIC EXAMINATION	An examination of a female that includes inspection of the external genitalia, a speculum exam, a vaginal exam, and a rectovaginal exam.
PROSTATECTOMY	The surgical removal of the prostate gland.
QUADRANTECTOMY	The surgical removal of the quarter of the breast that contains the lump.
RADICAL MASTECTOMY	The surgical removal of the breast, the underlying chest muscle, and the lymph nodes.
RECTOVAGINAL EXAMINATION	A procedure in which the physician places one finger in the vagina and another finger in the rectum. The fingers are then pressed together to check the condition of the walls of the rectum.
SIMPLE MASTECTOMY	The surgical removal of the breast and several lymph nodes.
SPECULUM EXAMINATION	A plastic or metal speculum is placed inside the vagina to hold the walls of the vagina open. The physician then checks for inflammation, growths, infections, and unusual discharge.
TESTICULAR SELF-EXAMINATION	Observation and palpation of the testes of a male to locate any lumps or tenderness.
THYROID EXAMINATION	The thyroid, located below the larynx, is palpated for any evidence of enlargement, lumps, or growths.
ULTRASOUND	An exam that involves the use of high-density sound waves to form images on a television screen. These images are reviewed by a physician.
URINALYSIS	An examination of a urine sample to check for infection, diabetes, or other abnormalities.

44. PHASES OF HUMAN SEXUAL RESPONSE

THE EXCITEMENT PHASE

Transition from a normal physical state to sexual arousal. This phase is characterized by erection of the penis in males, and vaginal moistening and enlargement of the clitoris in females. In both males and females, the heart rate and blood pressure increases and a "sex flush" resembling a rash may appear on the abdomen and breasts. The female breasts increase in size and the nipples become erect.

THE PLATEAU PHASE

During this phase, the breathing rate, heart rate, and blood pressure continue to increase. In males, the testes increase in size and a few drops of fluid from the Cowper's glands may emerge from the penis. In females, the clitoris retracts under the clitoral hood, the Bartholin's glands secrete fluid, the uterus elevates and increases in size, the inner two thirds of the vagina lengthens and expands, and the outer third of the vagina forms the orgasmic platform.

THE ORGASMIC PHASE

During this phase, a series of rhythmic contractions within the male penis, and similar contractions of the female's uterus occur. There is an increase in blood pressure, heart rate, and breathing rate in both males and females. In males, semen is expelled from the penis during ejaculation or orgasm.

THE RESOLUTION PHASE

This phase indicates a return to a nonarousal physical state. In both males and females, blood pressure, heart rate, and breathing begin to return to normal. In males, the penis quickly returns to its flaccid state and in females, the clitoris, breasts, labia, vagina, and uterus return to their unaroused state.

45. SEXUAL VARIATIONS AND PARAPHILIAS

Paraphilia is a sexual behavior or condition that focuses on sexual arousal or gratification through actions and fantasies that involve the use of objects or other people primarily for self-gratification.

ADULTERY   Sexual intercourse between a married person and an individual other than his or her legal spouse.

ANDROPHOBIA   Abnormal fear of men.

BESTIALITY   A sexual deviation in which a person engages in sexual relations with an animal.

BISEXUALITY   A sexual interest in both sexes.

COPROPHILIA   A sexual deviation in which sexual gratification is associated with the act of defecation; a morbid interest in feces.

EXHIBITIONISM   A sexual variance in which the individual, usually male, suffers from a compulsion to publicly expose his genitals.

FETISHISM   A sexual variance in which sexual gratification is achieved by means of an object, such as an article of clothing, that bears sexual symbolism for the individual.

FORNICATION   Sexual intercourse between two unmarried persons.

FROTTAGE   A sexual variance in which orgasm is induced by rubbing against an individual of the opposite sex, usually a stranger.

GERONTOSEXUALITY A sexual disorder in which a young person chooses an elderly person as the subject of his or her sexual interest.

HOMOSEXUALITY   Sexual attraction to, or sexual activity with, members of one's own sex.

INCEST   Sexual relations between close relatives, such as father and daughter, mother and son, or brother and sister.

KATASEXUALITY   Sexual behavior with a nonhuman partner.

MASOCHISM   A sexual variance in which an individual derives sexual gratification from having pain inflicted on him or her.

MASTURBATION   Self-stimulation of the genitals through manipulation.

NECROPHILIA   A sexual disorder in which an individual has a morbid sexual attraction to corpses.

NYMPHOMANIA   Excessive sexual desire in a woman.

PEDOPHILIA   A sexual deviation in which an adult engages in or desires sexual activity with a child.

POLYGAMY	The form of marriage in which a spouse of either sex has two or more mates at the same time.
PROSTITUTE	A person who engages in sexual relationships for payment.
PYROMANIA	A compulsion, usually sexually oriented, to start fires.
RAPE	Forcible sexual intercourse with a person who does not give consent, or who offers resistance.
SADISM	The achievement of sexual gratification by inflicting physical or psychological pain upon the sexual partner.
SATYRIASIS	Excessive sexual desire in a man.
SODOMY	A term, variously defined by law, to include sexual intercourse with animals and mouth-genital or anal intercourse between humans.
TRANSSEXUAL	A person having a desire, compulsion, or obsession to become a member of the opposite sex through surgical changes.
TRANSVESTITE	A person who derives sexual pleasure from wearing the garments of the opposite sex.
TROILISM	A sexual variance in which three people participate in a series of sexual practices.
VOYEURISM	A sexual variation in which a person achieves sexual gratification by observing others in the nude.

SECTION 3

DIET AND NUTRITION

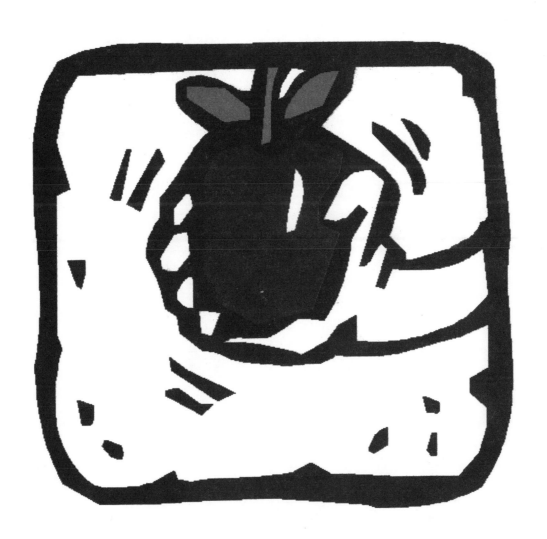

46. ESSENTIAL NUTRIENTS FOUND IN FOOD

CARBOHYDRATES   Made from carbon dioxide and water by green plants in the sunlight. Sugars, starches, and fiber are the most common carbohydrates.

FATS   Also known as lipids, and found in the bodies of animals and some vegetable oils (coconut, palm, and palm kernel).

PROTEINS   Vital organic substances made up of chains of the body's building blocks (amino acids), and found mainly in animal foods.

VITAMINS   Organic chemicals essential in small amounts for normal metabolism.

MINERALS   Inorganic elements that the body is unable to manufacture, but that are widely distributed in nature and have vital roles in metabolism.

WATER   The body's most essential nutrient, vital to every body function.

47. NUTRITIONAL FUNCTIONS AND SOURCES OF PROTEIN

FUNCTIONS OF PROTEINS

➡ Used mainly for building and maintaining all body tissues
➡ Enzyme, hormone, and antibody proteins help regulate body processes
➡ Used as an energy source to supplement carbohydrates and fats

SOURCES OF PROTEINS

➡ Animal sources (complete protein source)

meat	fish
poultry	eggs
milk	cheese
yogurt	

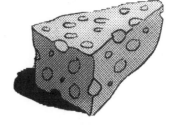

➡ Plant sources (incomplete protein source)

legumes	seeds
nuts	

48. NUTRITIONAL FUNCTIONS AND SOURCES OF CARBOHYDRATES

NUTRITIONAL FUNCTIONS OF CARBOHYDRATES

➡ The body's most important source of energy—calories
➡ Allow proteins to be used for building and repairing the body cells

SOURCES OF CARBOHYDRATES

vegetables	legumes
pasta	seeds
nuts	fruits
milk	sugar
syrup	molasses

49. NUTRITIONAL FUNCTIONS AND SOURCES OF FAT

NUTRITIONAL FUNCTIONS OF FAT

➡ An important source of calories
➡ Carries fat soluble vitamins (A, D, E, and K) into your blood
➡ Provides essential fatty acids
➡ Adds flavor to food
➡ Helps to satisfy hunger due to slower digestion
➡ Serves as a form of stored energy
➡ Protects vital organs from injury
➡ Insulates body from heat and cold

SOURCES OF FAT

➡ Visible fats

vegetable oil	meat/poultry
butter	margarine

➡ Hidden fats

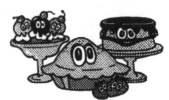

seed	nuts
eggs	ice cream
cheese	cream soups
sauces	cooking grease

50. NUTRITIONAL FUNCTIONS AND SOURCES OF CHOLESTEROL

NUTRITIONAL FUNCTIONS OF CHOLESTEROL

- ➡ Produces certain hormones
- ➡ Produces vitamin D (in the presence of sunlight)
- ➡ Produces the protective sheath around nerve fibers
- ➡ Makes bile acids that aid digestion

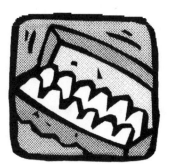

SOURCES OF CHOLESTEROL

- ➡ Human liver produces cholesterol
- ➡ Dietary Cholesterol:

Meat	Poultry
Fish	Eggs
Dairy Products	

51. NUTRITIONAL FUNCTIONS AND SOURCES OF VITAMINS

NUTRITIONAL FUNCTIONS OF VITAMINS

- ➡ Assist in the regulation of many body processes
- ➡ Work with enzymes by triggering chemical reactions which allow the digestion, absorption, metabolism, and use of other nutrients
- ➡ Speed up reactions that produce energy in body cells

NUTRITIONAL FUNCTIONS OF WATER-SOLUBLE VITAMINS

- ➡ C (ascorbic acid)—protects against infection, assists in healing of wounds, helps maintain strength and elasticity of blood vessels
- ➡ B_1 (thiamin)—changes glucose into energy or fat, helps prevent nervous irritability; necessary for good appetite
- ➡ B_2 (riboflavin)—transports hydrogen; is essential in the metabolism of carbohydrates, fats, and proteins; helps keep skin in healthy condition
- ➡ Niacin—hydrogen transport; important to maintenance of all body tissues; energy production
- ➡ B_6 (pyridoxine)—essential to amino acid and carbohydrate metabolism
- ➡ Pantothenic acid—functions in the breakdown and synthesis of carbohydrates, fats, and proteins; necessary for synthesis of some of the adrenal hormones

➠ Folacin (folic acid)—necessary for the production of RNA and DNA and normal red blood cells

➠ B_{12} (cyanocobalamin)—necessary for production of red blood cells and normal growth

NUTRITIONAL FUNCTIONS OF FAT-SOLUBLE VITAMINS

➠ Vitamin A—maintenance of epithelial tissue; strengthens tooth enamel and favors utilization of calcium and phosphorus in bone formation

➠ Vitamin D—promotes absorption and utilization of calcium and phosphorus; essential for normal bone and tooth development

➠ Vitamin E—May relate to oxidation and longevity, as well as protection against red blood cell destruction

➠ Vitamin K—Shortens blood-clotting time

SOURCES OF VITAMINS

Sources of Water-Soluble Vitamins

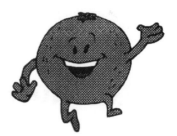

C (ascorbic acid)

citrus fruits	tomatoes
cabbage	broccoli
potatoes	peppers

B_1 (thiamin)

Whole-grain or enriched cereals

wheat germ	legumes
yeast	liver
nuts	

B_2 (riboflavin)

liver	green, leafy vegetables
milk	whole-grain cereal
eggs	enriched cereal
fish	cheese

Niacin

wheat germ	yeast
liver	eggs
fish	

B_6 (pyridoxine)

yeast	wheat bran
liver	wheat germ
meat	whole grains
fish	vegetables

Pantothenic acid

liver	whole-grain cereals
milk	whole-grain breads
yeast	green vegetables
kidney	wheat germ

Folacin (folic acid)

liver	green vegetables
nuts	orange juice

B_{12} (cyanocobalamin)

meat	liver
eggs	milk

Sources of Fat-Soluble Vitamins

Vitamin A

milk	dairy products
carrots	green vegetables
animal liver	

Vitamin D

beef	fish oils
butter	eggs
milk	sunlight

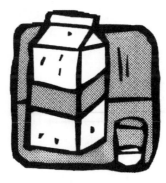

Vitamin E

yellow vegetable oils
wheat germ

Vitamin K

tomatoes	cabbage
eggs	spinach
liver	

Source: *Recommended Dietary Allowances*, 7th ed. Washington DC: National Academy of Sciences Publication.

52. NUTRITIONAL FUNCTIONS AND SOURCES OF ESSENTIAL MINERALS

NUTRITIONAL FUNCTIONS OF ESSENTIAL MINERALS

➡ Calcium (Ca)—building material of bones and teeth; regulation of body functions; heart muscle contraction, blood clotting

➡ Phosphorus (P)—combines with calcium to give rigidity to bones and teeth; essential in cell metabolism; helps to maintain proper acid-base balance of blood

➡ Iron (Fe)—component of the red blood cell's oxygen and carbon dioxide transport system; necessary for cellular respiration; important for use of energy in cells and for resistance to infection

➡ Iodine (I)—Essential component of the thyroid hormone, thyroxin, which controls the rate of cell oxidation; helps maintain proper water balance

➡ Sodium (Na)—regulates the fluid and acid-base balance in the body

➡ Chloride (Cl)—associated with sodium and its functions; a part of the gastric juice, hydrochloric acid; the chloride ion also functions in the starch-splitting system of saliva

➡ Potassium (K)—part of the system that controls the acid-base and liquid balances; thought to be an important enzyme activator in the use of amino acids

➡ Magnesium (Mg)—enzyme-activator related to carbohydrate metabolism

➡ Sulfur (S)—component of the hormone insulin and the sulfur amino acids; builds hair, nails, skin

➡ Manganese (Mn)—enzyme activator for systems related to carbohydrate, protein, and fat metabolism

➡ Copper (Cu)—essential ingredient in several respiratory enzymes; needed for development of red blood cells

➡ Zinc (Z)—component of many enzyme systems; and is an essential component of the pancreatic hormone insulin

➡ Cobalt (Co)—essential component of vitamin B_{12}

➡ Fluorine (F)—essential to normal bone and tooth development; excesses are undesirable

➡ Molybdenum (Mo)—essential for enzymes that make up uric acid

Source: Recommended Dietary Allowances, 7th ed. Washington DC: National Academy of Sciences Publication.

53. NUTRITIONAL FUNCTIONS OF WATER

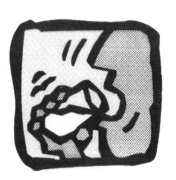

➠ Carries nutrients to the cell

➠ Transports wastes from the cell

➠ Lubricates the joints and mucous membranes

➠ Enables the body to swallow and digest foods

➠ Enables the body to eliminate wastes

➠ Cools the body down through the process of perspiration

➠ Prevents the buildup of internal heat

54. NUTRITIONAL FUNCTIONS AND SOURCES OF FIBER

NUTRITIONAL FUNCTIONS OF FIBER

➠ Helps to move waste through the digestive system

➠ Helps to prevent constipation

➠ Helps to prevent appendicitis

➠ Helps to protect the body from some cancers

➠ Helps to prevent heart disease

➠ Helps the body control diabetes

➠ Helps to lower cholesterol

➠ Assists in weight control (lower in fat and calories, less fiber is necessary to achieve a feeling of fullness)

SOURCES OF FIBER

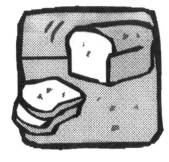

➠ fruits

➠ vegetables

➠ whole-grain products

55. U.S. RECOMMENDED DAILY DIETARY ALLOWANCES

Nutrient	Amount
Vitamin A	5,000 International Units (IU)
Vitamin C	60 milligrams (mg)
Thiamin	1.5 mg
Riboflavin	1.7 mg
Niacin	20 mg
Calcium	1.0 gram (g)
Iron	18 mg
Vitamin D	400 IU
Vitamin E	30 IU
Vitamin B6	2.0 mg
Folic Acid	0.4 mg
Vitamin B_{12}	6 micrograms (mcg)
Phosphorus	1.0 g
Iodine	150 mcg
Magnesium	400 mg
Zinc	15 mg
Copper	2 mg
Biotin	0.3 mg
Pantothenic Acid	10 mg

Source: Based on National Academy of Sciences, 1968 Recommended Daily Allowances.

56. U.S. DIETARY GUIDELINES FOR HEALTHY NUTRITION

DIETARY GUIDELINES FOR AMERICANS

➡ Eat a variety of foods

➡ Maintain healthy weight

➡ Choose a diet low in fat, saturated fat, and cholesterol

➡ Choose a diet with plenty of vegetables, fruits, and grain products

➡ Use sugars only in moderation

➡ Use salt and sodium only in moderation

➡ If you drink alcoholic beverages, do so in moderation

Source: Third Edition, 1990, U.S. Department of Agriculture, U.S. Department of Health and Human Services, Home and Garden Bulletin No. 232.

57. INFORMATION INCLUDED ON FOOD LABELS

➠ Name of the product

➠ Net quantity of contents

➠ Nutritional facts

➠ Ingredient list

➠ Name of manufacturer, packer, or distributor

➠ Address of manufacturer, packer, or distributor

➠ Name of the food

➠ Form of the food

➠ Quantity of the food in both pound and metric units

➠ Product dates (various dates may be used)

> Pull date—last recommended date of sale
> Quality assurance or freshness date—date for optimal food quality
> Pack date—date food was packaged or processed
> Expiration date—last day on which a product should be eaten

➠ Health claims (linking the effect of food to a health condition)

> Diet with enough calcium and lower risk of osteoporosis
> Diet low in fat and a reduced risk of some cancers
> Diet low in saturated fat and cholesterol and a reduced risk of coronary heart disease
> Diet rich in fiber and a reduced risk of some cancers
> Diet rich in fiber and a reduced risk of coronary heart disease
> Diet low in sodium and a reduced risk of high blood pressure
> Diet rich in fruits and vegetables and a reduced risk of some cancers

➠ Nutrient content claims (eleven terms relating to nutrients)

Free	Low
Reduced	Fewer
Lean	High
Less	More
Extra lean	Light
Good source	

➠ Other information that may appear on the food label

> Grades and standards
> Trademarks and copyrights
> Religious symbols
> Universal Product Code (UPC)
> Safe food handling instructions

58. NUTRITIONAL INFORMATION ON FOOD LABELS

SITUATIONS REQUIRING NUTRITIONAL LABELS

➠ When nutrients have been added during processing

➠ When a nutritional claim is made

➠ When dietary guidelines are present

NUTRITIONAL INFORMATION ON FOOD LABELS

➠ Serving size

➠ Servings per container

➠ Calories per serving

➠ Grams of protein, carbohydrate, and fat per serving

➠ Percent of U.S. Recommended Dietary Allowances (RDA) for protein and several vitamins and minerals

➠ Additional information may be included

      Milligrams of sodium

      Fat content

      Cholesterol content

      Fiber content

      Nutrient information when food is eaten with another food

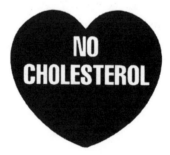

59. THE FOOD GUIDE PYRAMID

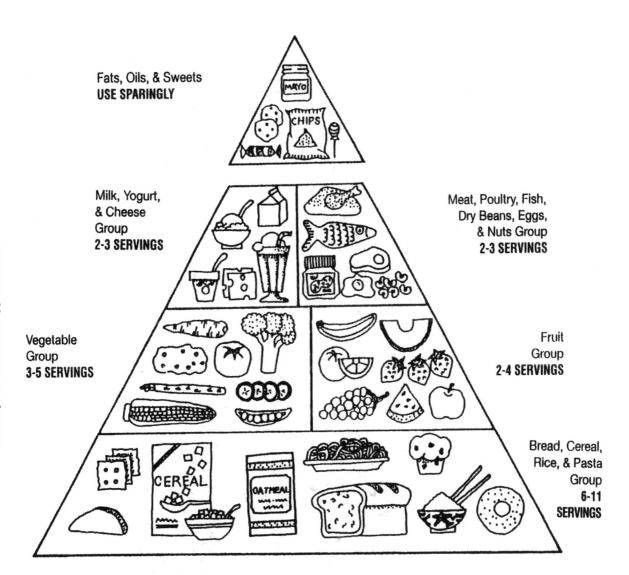

Fats, Oils, & Sweets
USE SPARINGLY

Milk, Yogurt,
& Cheese
Group
2-3 SERVINGS

Meat, Poultry, Fish,
Dry Beans, Eggs,
& Nuts Group
2-3 SERVINGS

Vegetable
Group
3-5 SERVINGS

Fruit
Group
2-4 SERVINGS

Bread, Cereal,
Rice, & Pasta
Group
**6-11
SERVINGS**

THE FOOD GUIDE PYRAMID
A Guide to Daily Food Choices

60. CLASSIFICATIONS OF VEGETARIANS

LACTO-OVO-VEGETARIAN (LACTOVARIAN)	Most common type of vegetarian; eats both dairy products and eggs.
LACTO-VEGETARIAN (LACTARIAN)	Eats dairy products but not eggs.
OVO-VEGETARIAN (OVARIAN)	Eats eggs but not dairy products.
PURE VEGETARIAN (VEGAN)	Does not eat dairy products, eggs, or any other animal product.
FRUITARIAN	Eats only plant food that can be harvested without killing plant.

61. COMMON CAUSES OF OVERWEIGHT AND OBESITY

➡ Burning too few calories through lack of physical exercise
➡ Taking in more calories than are burned
➡ Changes in metabolic rates with age
➡ Unhealthy eating habits
➡ Psychological factors
➡ Genetic inheritance
➡ The environment
➡ Social factors

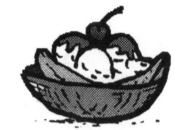

62. BENEFITS OF A REGULAR EXERCISE PROGRAM

➡ Burns calories
➡ Helps relieve stress
➡ Increases self-esteem
➡ Tones and builds muscles
➡ Promotes normal appetite
➡ Promotes loss of body fat
➡ Helps increase metabolic rate
➡ Gives body a firm, lean shape

63. NUMBER OF CALORIES BURNED BY 150-POUND PERSON IN VARIOUS PHYSICAL ACTIVITIES

Activity	Gross Energy Spent in Calories Per Hour
Rest and light activities	*50–200*
Lying down or sleeping	80
Sitting	100
Driving an automobile	120
Domestic work	180
Moderate activity	*200–350*
Bicycling (5-1/2 mph)	210
Walking (2-1/2 mph)	210
Gardening	220
Canoeing (2-1/2 mph)	230
Golf	250
Lawn mowing (power mower)	250
Fencing	300
Rowboating (2-1/2 mph)	300
Swimming(1/4 mph)	300
Walking (3-1/4 mph)	300
Badminton	350
Horseback riding (trotting)	350
Square dancing	350
Volleyball	350
Roller skating	350
Vigorous activity	*over 350*
Table tennis	360
Ditch digging (hand shovel)	400
Ice skating (10 mph)	400
Wood chopping or sawing	400
Tennis	420
Water skiing	480
Hill climbing (100 feet per hour)	490
Skiing (10 mph)	600
Squash and handball	600
Cycling (13 mph)	660
Scull rowing (race)	840
Running (10 mph)	900

Source: President's Council on Physical Fitness and Sports, *Exercise and Weight Control.* Washington, DC: U.S. Government Printing Office, 1979.

64. COMMON EATING DISORDERS

According to the American Anorexia/Bulimia Association, Inc., more than 5 million Americans suffer from eating disorders.

ANOREXIA NERVOSA — Typically involves irrational fear of becoming obese, and results in severe weight loss due to self-starvation; may include bingeing and purging behavior.

BULIMIA NERVOSA — Typically involves extremely restrictive dieting and regular and repeated binge eating, followed by self-induced vomiting, purging through abuse of laxatives, diuretics, or enemas, or excessive physical activity.

COMPULSIVE OVEREATING — Characterized by uncontrollable eating despite lack of hunger; often includes a preoccupation with food and body image.

BINGE-EATING DISORDER — Characterized by regular and repeated binge-eating episodes; does not include purging or other behaviors.

65. SYMPTOMS AND CAUSES OF ANOREXIA AND BULIMIA

SYMPTOMS OF ANOREXIA AND BULIMIA

- Feelings of shame, loneliness
- Being secretive about weight
- Avoidance of mirrors
- Rituals including food
- Need to be perfect
- Prior sexual abuse
- Difficulty relaxing
- Need to exercise
- Need for control
- Good student
- Use of food for emotional comfort
- Preoccupation with appearance
- Inability to recognize hunger
- Lack of emotional reactions
- Compulsive behaviors
- Feeling of depression
- Being secretive about food
- Fear of growing up
- Suicide attempts
- Denial of hunger
- Excellent athlete

CAUSES OF ANOREXIA AND BULIMIA

- Low self-esteem
- Fear of becoming fat
- Feelings of helplessness
- Need to reduce stress and anxiety
- Inability to cope with typical problems
- Possible neuroendocrine system irregularities
- Fear of growing up and becoming independent
- Need to gain a sense of control in some area of life
- Parents who are overly concerned with child's physical appearance
- Involvement in activities that emphasize thinness:

Modeling	Dancing
Gymnastics	Wrestling
Long-distance running	

66. INTERESTING DIET AND NUTRITION FACTS

➠ An average man weighing approximately 150 pounds will have to eat about 50 tons of food during his lifetime to maintain his weight

➠ One-third of adults in the United States are overweight, and one-half have cholesterol levels above the desired 200 mg/dl level

➠ Commercials shown during the top-rated television shows feature food products more than any other kind of product

➠ Each person in the United States eats almost four pounds of preservatives and artificial flavorings and colorings each year

➠ Every day in the United States, people consume

> 200 million pounds of fresh fruit and vegetables,
> 50 million pounds of sugar,
> 47 million hot dogs,
> 170 million eggs,
> 12.5 million pounds of cheese,
> 12 million chickens,
> 7 million pounds of margarine,
> 3 million pounds of butter,
> 3 million gallons of ice milk and ice cream,
> 1.2 million bushels of potatoes, and
> 363 thousand square yards of pizza

➠ About 65% of the sugar Americans consume is in processed foods

➠ The body can eliminate only 100 mg of cholesterol gained from foods each day; anything more than that begins to clog the arteries

➠ Removing one tablespoon of fat from the daily diet can help most people lose up to 10 pounds per year

➠ A cup of skim milk contains more calcium (320 mg) than a cup of whole milk (290 mg)

➠ Most 12-ounce cans of cola contain water, caffeine, carbonation, about 9 teaspoons of sugar, and no other nutrients

➠ In 1202, King John of England proclaimed the first English food law, the Assize of Bread, which prohibited adulteration of bread with such ingredients as ground peas or beans

SECTION 4

CONSUMER HEALTH

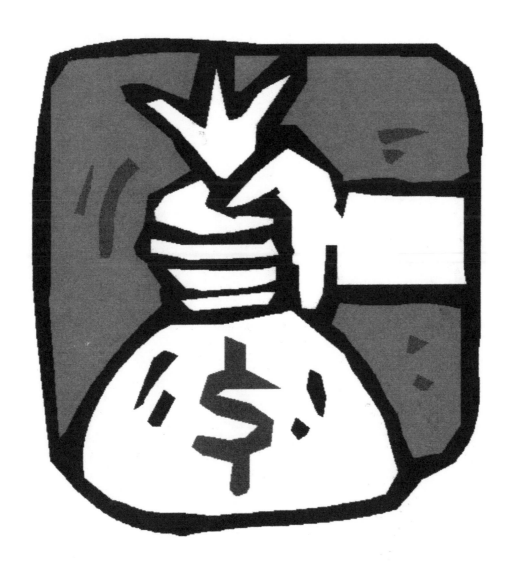

67. ADVANTAGES OF BEING A WISE CONSUMER

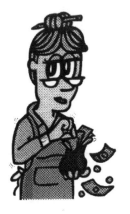

➠ Wise consumers save money. They are able to make the best purchase for the least amount of money.

➠ Wise consumers protect their health. They are not persuaded to buy products and services that are worthless or harmful.

➠ Wise consumers develop a high level of self-confidence. They are able to speak up for their rights if they feel they have been treated unfairly.

68. CONSUMER BILL OF RIGHTS

Introduced in 1962 by President John F. Kennedy:

➠ The right to safety. Consumers are protected from dangerous products.

➠ The right to be informed. Consumers are protected from misleading advertising.

➠ The right to choose. Consumers have the right to make their own choices.

➠ The right to be heard. Consumers can speak out when they are not satisfied.

President Richard Nixon added:

➠ The right to redress. Consumers have the right to have any wrong done to them corrected.

President Gerald Ford added:

➠ The right to consumer education

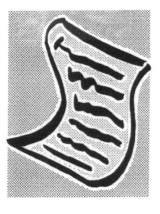

69. FACTORS THAT INFLUENCE BUYING DECISIONS

PRICE Unit pricing information on store shelves assists consumers with product comparison.

CONVENIENCE Labor-saving features of products can affect what consumers buy and how much they pay.

FAMILY AND FRIENDS People who are special to us can influence our buying decisions.

QUALITY Guarantees and label information can assist the consumer with purchasing decisions.

ADVERTISING Persuasion techniques used by advertisers can influence consumers to purchase products.

70. ADVERTISING PERSUASION TECHNIQUES

NOSTALGIA Plain folks, back-to-nature, just the way Grandma used to make it, back in the good old days.

BANDWAGON Everyone who is anyone is buying this product. Don't be the only one without it. Don't be left out!

TRANSFER/FANTASY Superheros, white knights, green giants, super athletes, beautiful people, or rich people are featured. Advertisers hope that the consumer will transfer these qualities to the products and themselves, and purchase the product.

HUMOR People tend to remember an ad if it makes them laugh, and may purchase the product because of the positive association with it.

SENSE APPEAL Sounds or pictures that appeal to the senses are featured.

STATISTICS People tend to be impressed with "facts" and statistics, even if they have little or no meaning.

TESTIMONIAL Important or well-known people testify that they use the product, and so should you.

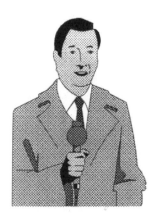

Source: Toner, Patricia Rizzo, *Consumer Health and Safety Activities*. West Nyack, NY: The Center for Applied Research in Education, 1993.

71. HEALTH PRODUCTS COMMONLY SUSCEPTIBLE TO FRAUD

FDA's List of the Top Health Frauds:

FRAUDULENT ARTHRITIS PRODUCTS

Copper bracelets, Chinese herbal remedies, large doses of vitamins, and snake or bee venom have no proven value. Because the symptoms of arthritis go into remission periodically, individuals who try these unproven remedies may associate the remedy with the remission.

SPURIOUS CANCER CLINICS

These clinics promise miracle cures. Treatments are unproven and use ineffective substances and vitamins and minerals. People who go to these clinics often abandon legitimate cancer treatments. This is particularly tragic in the case of young children, because some of their cancers (such as leukemia or Hodgkin's disease) are highly curable through legitimate treatment.

BOGUS AIDS CURES

Victims of incurable diseases such as AIDS, are especially vulnerable to the promises of charlatans.

INSTANT WEIGHT-LOSS SCHEMES

Unfortunately, there is no quick way to lose weight. Some of the gimmicks used in instant weight-loss plans have included skin patches, herbal capsules, grapefruit diet pills, and Chinese magic weight-loss earrings.

FRAUDULENT SEXUAL AIDS

The FDA says no nonprescription drug ingredients have been proven safe or effective as aphrodisiacs, and has acted to ban these products. Although male sex hormones, available by prescription, do influence libido and sexual performance, they have potentially serious side effects, and should be used only under a physician's supervision.

QUACK BALDNESS REMEDIES AND OTHER APPEAR-ANCE MODIFIERS

The FDA has acted to ban the sale of any nonprescription hair cream, lotion, or other external product claiming to grow hair or prevent baldness. None of these products has been shown to work. The FDA has not evaluated safety and effectiveness data for any drug's use as a wrinkle remover. So-called breast developers have also been used by millions of women who want larger breasts, but experts point out that these devices do not increase breast size.

FALSE NUTRITIONAL SCHEMES

Various food products (such as bee pollen, over-the-counter herbal remedies, and wheat germ capsules) are promoted as sure-fire cures for various diseases. Though usually not harmful, these products have not been proven beneficial.

UNPROVEN USE OF MUSCLE STIMULATORS

The FDA considers the promotion of muscle stimulators to perform face lifts, to reduce breast size, to remove cellulite, and for the removal of wrinkles to be fraudulent.

72. METHODS OF RECOGNIZING FRAUDULENT PRACTICES OR PRODUCTS

Quackery often follows certain patterns. If the answer to any of the following questions is yes, be wary of fraud:

➡ Does the promoter of the product or service claim to be battling the medical profession, which is supposed to be trying to suppress the wonderful discovery?

➡ Does he or she maintain that surgery, x-rays, or medication prescribed by reputable physicians will do more harm than good?

➡ Is the remedy sold from door to door by a self-styled "health advisor," or advertised at public lectures?

➡ Is the product promoted in a sensational magazine or by a faith healer's group?

➡ Does the seller use scare tactics, predicting all sorts of harmful consequences if you do not use the product?

➡ Is the product or service offered as a "secret remedy"?

➡ Does the promoter show testimonials to demonstrate the wonders that the product or service has performed for others?

➡ Is the product or service claiming to be good for a vast array of illnesses, or guaranteed to provide a quick cure?

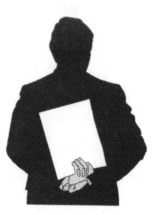

73. AGENCIES THAT PROTECT CONSUMERS

BETTER BUSINESS BUREAU (BBB)	Nonprofit group sponsored by private businesses that provide information on products and services.
CONSUMER AFFAIRS OFFICES	State, county, and city offices that assist consumers with product and service complaints. They offer a large selection of educational materials.
PRIVATE CONSUMER GROUPS	Individual consumers who work together in support of consumer interests.
MEDIA PROGRAMS	Help lines for consumer issues provided through television, radio, newspapers, and so forth.
PROFESSIONAL LICENSING BOARDS	Assist consumers with issues concerning physicians and dentists.
SMALL-CLAIMS COURT	Available locally and deals with claims that are between $100 and $3,000.

74. BETTER BUSINESS BUREAU SERVICES

The Better Business Bureau (BBB) is a nonprofit organization sponsored by private businesses.

Better Business Bureau services:

➡ Provides general information on products and services of local businesses and organizations

➡ Provides reliability reports and background information on local businesses and organizations

➡ Provides records of companies' complaint-handling performances

➡ Attempts to settle consumer complaints against local businesses

➡ Accepts written complaints and contacts firms on behalf of the consumer

➡ Handles false advertising cases for consumers

Additional information is available by contacting:

COUNCIL OF BETTER BUSINESS BUREAUS, INC.
4200 Wilson Blvd., Suite 800
Arlington, VA 22203-1804
Phone: (703) 276-0100
Fax: (703) 525-8277
http://www.bbb.org/

75. FEDERAL GOVERNMENT AGENCIES THAT DEAL WITH HEALTH-RELATED PRODUCTS AND SERVICES

THE CONSUMER PRODUCT SAFETY COMMISSION (CPSC)

Develops and enforces safety standards for products from household appliances and power tools to toys and children's sleepwear. The CPSC has the power to ban or order the recall of unacceptably hazardous products. The CPSC also regulates packaging of prescriptions and over-the-counter medicines. Information is available from the Consumer Product Safety Commission, Bethesda, Maryland 20207. Web site: http://www.cpsc.gov

THE CONSUMER INFORMATION CENTER (CIC)

Distributes consumer information published by the federal government. Free copies of the Catalog of Consumer Information is available from the Consumer Information Center, Pueblo, Colorado, 81009 or by e-mail at catalog.pueblo@gsa.gov Web site: http://www.cic.gov

THE FOOD AND DRUG ADMINIS- TRATION (FDA)

Created to protect consumers against unsafe and ineffective health products. Enforces the Food, Drug, and Cosmetic Act, which bans false and misleading statements on drug labels; requires that active ingredients be listed on labels; demands that all manufactured foods, drugs, and cosmetics be proved safe, and drugs be proved effective before they can be marketed; requires that drug labels list side effects; and permits the immediate recall of hazardous drugs. Also judges the safety and effectiveness of certain medical devices, such as x-ray equipment, pacemakers, and artificial heart valves. Information is available from the Food and Drug Administration, Rockville, Maryland, 20857.

Phone: 1-800-532-4440 (in the Washington, D.C., area,
    please call 301-827-4420)
Fax: 301-443-9767
E-Mail: execsec@oc.fda.gov
Web site: http://www.fda.gov

THE FOOD SAFETY AND INSPECTION SERVICE (FSIS)

A division of the Department of Agriculture that ensures that meat, poultry, and the products made from them are safe, wholesome, and labeled properly. Provides information and educational materials on food safety and purchasing. Information available from the Information Division, Food Safety and Inspection Service, Department of Agriculture, Washington, DC 20250.

THE FEDERAL TRADE COMMISSION (FTC)

Protects consumers against injuries that could result from false advertising and unfair selling practices, including the omission of important information from product labels. Information is available from the Office of the Secretary, Federal Trade Commission, Washington, DC 20580.
Web site: http://www.ftc.gov

THE BUREAU OF CONSUMER PROTECTION OF THE FEDERAL AVIATION ADMINISTRATION (FAA) — Handles complaints against airlines. Information is available from the Bureau of Consumer Protection, Federal Aviation Administration, Washington, DC 20428.
Web site: http://www.faa.gov

THE UNITED STATES POSTAL SERVICE — Guards the public against the sale of fraudulent products by mail.
Web site: http://www.usps.gov

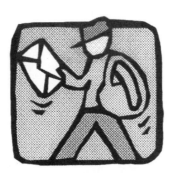

76. STEPS TO RESOLVE CONSUMER PROBLEMS

➡ Identify the problem and a method of resolution

➡ Compile documentation that will substantiate the claim (canceled check, sales receipt, etc.)

➡ Attempt to resolve the problem with the individual who sold the product or performed the service

➡ Attempt to resolve the problem with the supervisor or manager

➡ Write a letter to the company president or the director of consumer affairs of the company

➡ Contact a consumer information agency for assistance

77. ITEMS TO INCLUDE IN A CONSUMER COMPLAINT LETTER

When it becomes necessary to write a letter of complaint to a company, the letter should include the following:

➡ The name and title of the person to whom you are writing

➡ The name of the product and serial or model number, or type of service provided

➡ The date and location of the product or service

➡ A statement of the problem or complaint

➡ A request for a resolution to the problem in a reasonable amount of time

➡ The consumer's address and phone number

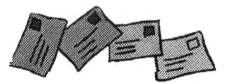

78. GUIDELINES FOR CHOOSING A HEALTH PROFESSIONAL

First check your health plan to see if it restricts you to using its own list of approved doctors.

If you can choose any doctor you want, but need help in finding one, do the following:

➥ Ask family members and friends for their recommendations.

➥ Be sure the doctor is licensed and in good standing.

➥ Contact the nearest county medical association for a list or brochure with names of board-certified doctors in your area.

➥ Call a nearby hospital for information on its doctors and other health professionals.

Before making your first appointment, ask the receptionist these questions:

➥ Is the doctor accepting new patients?

➥ How long has the doctor been in practice?

➥ How far in advance must you make an appointment?

➥ What hospital does the doctor use?

➥ Does the office accept your health insurance plan?

➥ What is the fee for an office visit?

After your office visit, ask yourself these questions:

➥ Are staff members friendly and professional?

➥ Is the facility pleasant and clean?

➥ Are educational materials or programs available for patients?

➥ Does the doctor appear to be a caring person?

➥ Does he or she provide enough time and attention for a thorough examination?

➥ Does he or she listen well and encourage patients to ask questions?

➥ Does he or she explain things in a way that is easy to understand?

➥ Does he or she encourage the practice of preventive medicine?

➥ Does he or she encourage patients to take part in their own health care?

79. TYPES OF PHYSICIANS

ALLERGIST	Allergy specialist.
ANESTHESIOLOGIST	Physician who administers anesthetics during surgery.
CARDIOLOGIST	Heart specialist.
DERMATOLOGIST	Skin specialist.
ENDOCRINOLOGIST	Specialist in glandular disorders.
GASTROENTEROLOGIST	Specialist in the disorders of the digestive tract.
HEMATOLOGIST/ ONCOLOGIST	Blood and cancer specialist.
MEDICAL INTERNIST	Physician practicing nonsurgical, adult medicine.
NEPHROLOGIST	Kidney specialist.
NEUROLOGIST	Specialist in disorders of brain and nervous system.
OBSTETRICIAN/ GYNECOLOGIST	Physician dealing with childbirth and women's diseases.
OPHTHALMOLOGIST	Eye specialist.
ORTHOPEDIC SURGEON	Specialist who performs surgery on bones and joints.
OTOLARYNGOLOGIST	Specialist in the treatment of eye, ear, nose, and throat.
OTOLOGIST	Ear specialist.
PATHOLOGIST	Specialist in the causes of death.
PEDIATRICIAN	Specialist in the treatment of children.
PLASTIC SURGEON	Specialist in the treatment of skin and soft tissue deformities.
PODIATRIST	Foot specialist.
PSYCHIATRIST	Physician specializing in the treatment of mental illness.
RADIOLOGIST	Specialist in the use of x-ray and radium therapy.
RHEUMATOLOGIST	Specialist in disorders involving connective tissue such as joints and muscles.
THORACIC SURGEON	Specialist in surgery on the chest and lungs.
VASCULAR SURGEON	Specialist in surgery on the heart and blood vessels.
UROLOGIST	Specialist in the treatment of the urinary tract.

80. TYPES OF DENTAL SPECIALISTS

ENDODONTIST   Specializes in the prevention, diagnosis, and treatment of diseases and injuries that affect the root of the tooth and related tissue.

ORAL SURGEON   Specializes in the surgical removal of teeth and the surgical correction of mouth disorders.

ORTHODONTIST   Specializes in the development, prevention, and correction of irregularities of the teeth.

PEDODONTIST   Specializes in the treatment of children's dental problems.

PERIODONTIST   Specializes in the treatment and prevention of gum disease.

81. QUESTIONS TO ASK ABOUT PRESCRIPTION DRUGS

The American Heart Association recommends that consumers ask their physician the following questions before taking a prescription medicine.

➧ Why is the medication being prescribed?

➧ What is the name of the medicine?

➧ Does it have a generic form (effective but cheaper)?

➧ How should I take it—when, how often, and how long?

➧ Are printed instructions available?

➧ What are the benefits and side effects of this medicine?

➧ What food or drink restrictions should I know about?

➧ Is the dosage the lowest possible level for me but still effective?

➧ Is it compatible with all other medications I'm taking?

82. SAFETY MEASURES FOR STORING AND HANDLING MEDICINES

The Food and Drug Administration (FDA) recommends the following safety measures for the storing and handling of medicines:

➡ Date all over-the-counter drugs when purchased

➡ Buy medicines and health supplies in realistic quantities—only enough to meet immediate needs

➡ Store all drugs out of the reach of small children

➡ Read the label carefully, and observe all warnings

➡ Do not give or take an unlabeled medicine

➡ Do not give or take medicine in the dark

➡ Be attentive when measuring drugs

➡ Do not take multiple drugs at the same time without first consulting a physician

➡ Discard any old or leftover drugs

➡ Flush discarded drugs down the toilet, and rinse out empty containers before discarding

83.   BASICS FOR THE HOME MEDICINE CHEST

Nondrug Items	Drug Items
Adhesive tape	Analgesic (such as aspirin)
Bandaids—in assorted sizes	Antacid
Cotton balls	Antidiarrhetic
Cotton-tipped applicators	Antiseptic
Dosage spoon	Burn salve or ointment
Elastic bandage	Calamine lotion
Eye cup	Cortisone cream
First-aid manual	Cough syrup
Gauze pads and rolls	Decongestant
Heating pad	Ipecac
Hot water bottle	Petroleum jelly
Humidifier	
Ice bag or freezable cold compress	
Scissors—small size with blunt end	
Thermometer	
Tweezers	

SECTION 5

FIRST AID AND SAFETY

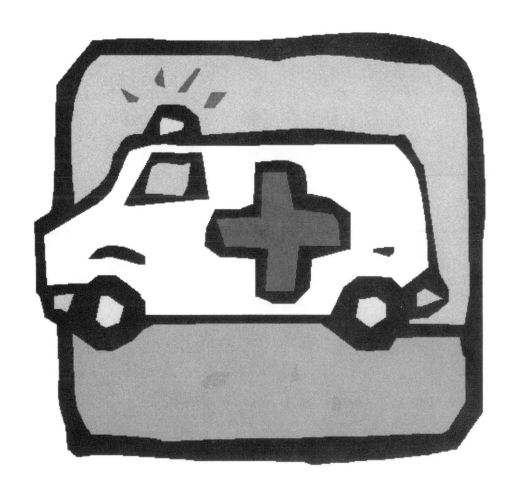

84. FIRST-AID PRIORITIES

According to the American Red Cross, it is important to remain calm, act quickly, and apply the following basic first-aid action principles in the event of an emergency:

SURVEY THE SCENE

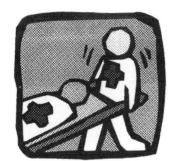

➠ Check to see if the situation is safe

➠ Look for clues as to what happened

➠ Check for a medical alert tag

➠ Check for other victims

➠ Ask bystanders for assistance

SURVEY THE VICTIM

➠ Check for an open airway

➠ Check to see if the victim is breathing

➠ Check circulation by checking for a pulse

PHONE THE EMERGENCY MEDICAL SERVICES (EMS) FOR ASSISTANCE

➠ EMS should be contacted when there is a life-threatening condition that requires the assistance of a trained medical professional.

85. WHAT TO REPORT WHEN PLACING AN EMERGENCY PHONE CALL

The American Red Cross recommends that the following information be given to emergency medical personnel when placing a 9-1-1 call:

➠ The location of the emergency (exact address, city or town, nearby intersections, landmarks, name of building, floor, apartment or room number)

➠ The telephone number from which the call is being made

➠ The caller's name

➠ What happened

➠ The number of victims

➠ The condition of the victim(s)

➠ The first aid being given

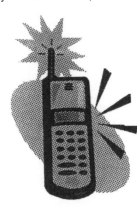

86. SIGNALS OF BREATHING EMERGENCIES

➡ Unusually slow or rapid breathing

➡ Unusually deep or shallow breaths

➡ Gasping for breath

➡ Wheezing, gurgling, or making high-pitched noises

➡ Skin is unusually moist

➡ Skin has a flushed, pale, or bluish appearance

➡ Shortness of breath

➡ Dizziness or lightheaded feeling

➡ Pain in chest or tingling in hands or feet

87. CAUSES AND PREVENTION OF CHOKING

According to the American Red Cross, choking is a common injury than can lead to death:

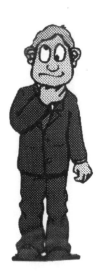

CAUSES OF CHOKING

➡ Trying to swallow large pieces of poorly chewed food

➡ Drinking alcohol before or during meals. (Alcohol dulls the nerves that help you swallow.)

➡ Wearing dentures. Dentures make it difficult to sense the size of food when chewing and swallowing.

➡ Talking excitedly or laughing while eating, or eating too fast

➡ Walking, playing, or running with objects in the mouth

PREVENTION OF CHOKING

➡ Don't leave small objects, such as buttons, coins, and beads, within an infant's reach

➡ Have children sit in a high chair or at a table while they eat

➡ Do not let children eat too fast

➡ Give infants soft food that they do not have to chew

➡ Make sure that toys are too large to be swallowed

➡ Do not give infants and young children foods like nuts, grapes, popcorn, and raw vegetables

➡ Make sure that toys have no small parts that could be pulled off

➡ Cut foods a child can choke on easily, such as hot dogs, into small pieces

88. FIRST AID FOR CHOKING

FIRST AID FOR CONSCIOUS CHOKING VICTIM

If the person is unable to cough, speak, or breathe:

→ Stand behind victim

→ Wrap arms around victim's waist

→ Place thumb side of fist against middle of victim's abdomen, just above the navel

→ Grasp fist with other hand

→ Give quick upwards thrusts

→ Repeat until object is coughed up or person becomes unconscious

FIRST AID FOR UNCONSCIOUS CHOKING VICTIM

→ With victim's head tilted back and chin lifted, pinch the nose shut

→ Give two slow breaths. Breathe into victim until chest gently rises

→ Check for a pulse

→ If pulse is present but person is still not breathing, give one slow breath about every 5 seconds for one minute. Recheck pulse and breathing

→ Continue rescue breathing as long as a pulse is present but person is not breathing

Source: American Red Cross Staff, *American Red Cross Community First Aid & Safety*. St. Louis, MO: Mosby-Yearbook, Inc., 1993.

89. SIGNS OF A HEART ATTACK

According to the American Red Cross, the following symptoms could signal a heart attack:

PERSISTENT CHEST PAIN OR DISCOMFORT	Victim has persistent pain or pressure in the chest that is not relieved by resting, changing position, or oral medication. Pain may range from discomfort to an unbearable crushing sensation.
BREATHING DIFFICULTY	Victim's breathing is noisy. Victim feels short of breath. Victim's breathing is faster than normal.
CHANGES IN PULSE RATE	Pulse may be faster or slower than normal, or it may be irregular.
SKIN APPEARANCE	Victim's skin may be pale or bluish in color. Victim's face may be moist, or victim may sweat profusely.

90. FIRST AID FOR A HEART ATTACK

➡ Recognize the signals of a heart attack

➡ Persuade the victim to stop activity and rest

➡ Help the victim to rest comfortably

➡ Try to obtain information about the victim's condition

➡ Comfort the victim

➡ Call the local emergency number for help

➡ Assist with medication, if prescribed

➡ Monitor the victim's condition

➡ Give CPR if the victim is not breathing and has no pulse

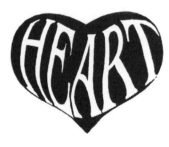

91. CARDIOPULMONARY RESUSCITATION (CPR)

According to the American Red Cross, CPR increases a cardiac arrest victim's chances of survival by keeping the brain supplied with oxygen until the victim can get medical care. Without CPR, the brain begins to die in as few as four minutes. The following procedure is recommended:

➡ Roll victim onto back, if necessary

➡ Find hand compression position in the center of breastbone
>   Locate notch where lower ribs meet breastbone
>   Place heel of the hand on the breastbone
>   Place other hand on top of the first
>   Keep fingers off chest

➡ Position shoulders over hands, lock elbows, and compress victim's chest 15 times using a smooth, even rhythm

➡ Hands should stay in contact with chest at all times

➡ Give 2 full breaths using head-tilt/chin-lift method
>   Pinch nose shut
>   Make a tight seal around outside of victim's mouth with your mouth
>   Watch for chest to rise and fall

➡ Do three more sets of 15 compressions and 2 breaths

➡ Recheck pulse and breathing for about 5 seconds

➡ If there is no pulse, continue sets of 15 compressions and 2 breaths until another trained person takes over

92. TYPES OF OPEN WOUNDS

CONTUSION (BRUISE, CHARLEY HORSE)	Damage to soft tissues and blood vessels causes bleeding under the skin. Tissues discolor and swell.
ABRASION (SCRAPE, ROAD RASH, RUG BURN, STRAWBERRY)	Most common type of wound. Caused by skin that has been scraped away. Painful, and can become easily infected.
INCISION/ LACERATION (CUT)	May have jagged or smooth edges. Nerves, large blood vessels, and other soft tissue can become damaged. Usually bleeds freely.
AVULSION	A cut in which soft tissue is partially or completely torn away. Characterized by heavy bleeding.
PUNCTURE	A wound caused when a pointed object, such as a nail, pierces the skin. Because punctures do not bleed a lot, infection is common.

93. TECHNIQUES TO CONTROL SEVERE BLEEDING

The American Red Cross recommends the following techniques to control external bleeding:

DIRECT PRESSURE   Place direct pressure on the wound with a dressing such as a sterile gauze pad or any clean cloth. Using a dressing will help keep the wound free from germs. Place a hand over the pad and press firmly.

ELEVATION   Elevate the injured part above the level of the heart if you do not suspect a broken bone.

PRESSURE BANDAGE   Apply a pressure bandage to hold the pad or cloth in place.

PRESSURE POINTS   If bleeding cannot be controlled, put pressure on the nearby artery.

Monitor the victim closely for signals that the condition is getting worse. Care for shock, if necessary.

94. SYMPTOMS OF AND FIRST AID FOR INTERNAL BLEEDING

SYMPTOMS OF INTERNAL BLEEDING

➡ Bruising or discolored skin in the injured area

➡ Soft tissues that are tender, swollen, or hard

➡ Anxiety or restlessness

➡ Fast, weak pulse

➡ Fast breathing

➡ Skin that feels cool or moist or looks pale or bluish

➡ Nausea and vomiting

➡ Strong thirst

➡ Decrease in level of consciousness

FIRST AID FOR INTERNAL BLEEDING

➡ Bruise—apply ice or a cold pack to help reduce pain and swelling

➡ For a more severe internal injury, call EMS immediately. While waiting for help:

Monitor breathing
Do no further harm, and reassure the victim
Help the victim rest in a comfortable position
Maintain the normal body temperature

Source: American Red Cross Staff, *American Red Cross Standard First Aid.* St. Louis, MO: Mosby-Year Book, Inc., 1991.

95. SYMPTOMS OF AND FIRST AID FOR SHOCK

SYMPTOMS OF SHOCK

➧ Dizziness and/or nausea

➧ Fatigue and/or weakness

➧ Thirst

➧ Scared or restless appearance

➧ Weak and rapid pulse

➧ Cool and clammy skin

➧ Sweating

➧ Dilated pupils

➧ Shallow and rapid breathing

➧ Shaking or shivering

➧ Pale skin

➧ Bluish lips and fingernails

FIRST AID FOR SHOCK

➧ Victim should lie down to reduce the stress on the body and to slow down any progression of the effects of shock

➧ Control any external bleeding

➧ Maintain the victim's normal body temperature

➧ Reassure the victim

➧ Elevate the legs about 12 inches, unless you suspect head, neck, or back injuries, or there is the possibility of broken bones involving the hips or legs

➧ Administer no food or drink, despite the probability of thirst

➧ Call EMS immediately. Shock victims require immediate medical care.

96. TYPES OF BURNS

According to the American Red Cross, burns are classified by their source and their depth.

FIRST-DEGREE BURNS	Involve only the top layer of skin. The skin is red and dry, the area may swell, and the burn is usually painful. Most sunburns are first-degree burns.
SECOND-DEGREE BURNS	Deeper than first-degree burns. Burned skin will look red and have blisters. The skin may appear wet if the blisters are open. The burned skin may look mottled. Usually painful, the area often swells, and scarring may occur.
THIRD-DEGREE BURNS	Extend through the skin and into the structures below the skin. These burns may look brown or charred. Can be extremely painful, or may be relatively painless if the burn destroyed the nerve endings in the skin. Scarring may be severe, and these burns may be life-threatening.

97. FIRST AID FOR BURNS

➡ Remove the victim from the source of the burn

➡ Use large amounts of cool water to cool the burn

➡ Do not use ice or ice water

➡ Use dry, sterile dressings or clean cloth to cover the burn to keep out air and reduce pain, and to help prevent infection

➡ Treat victim for shock

➡ Care for small first-degree burns as follows:

    Wash the area with soap and water
    Keep the area clean
    Apply an antibiotic ointment
    Watch for infection

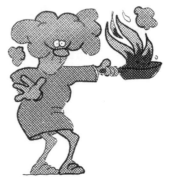

98. FIRST AID FOR FRACTURES, DISLOCATIONS, SPRAINS, AND STRAINS

Since it is often difficult to tell whether an injury is a fracture, dislocation, sprain, or strain, always treat the injury as a fracture by following these basic procedures:

➡ Do not move the victim unless he or she is in a dangerous situation

➡ Controlling any severe bleeding is a priority

➡ Treatment for shock

➡ Immobilize the suspected fracture by splinting the area above and below the joint

➡ Splint only if it does not cause additional pain and discomfort

➡ Splint the injury in the position in which it was found

➡ Monitor circulation before and after splinting

➡ Elevate area after splinting

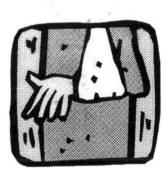

99. WAYS POISONING MAY OCCUR

A poison is any substance—solid, liquid, or gas—that causes injury or death when introduced into the body. The four ways that poisoning can occur:

INGESTION   The poison can be taken by mouth.

INHALATION   Poisoning can result from breathing in toxic fumes.

ABSORPTION   The poison can come into contact with the body and be absorbed through the skin.

INJECTION   The poison can enter the body by way of an animal or insect bite or sting, or be injected by a hypodermic needle.

100. SIGNALS OF AND FIRST AID FOR POISONING

SWALLOWED POISONS

Signals

Nausea	Vomiting
Diarrhea	Chest/abdominal pain
Breathing difficulty	Sweating
Loss of consciousness	Seizures
Burns around the mouth	Evidence of empty containers

First Aid

Call poison control center or EMS immediately.
Care for shock and monitor breathing.

INHALED POISONS

Signals

Dizziness	Headache
Breathing difficulty	Pale or bluish skin

First Aid

Remove victim from poisonous environment without putting yourself in danger.
Call for emergency assistance.
Monitor victim's breathing.

ABSORBED POISONS

Signals

Skin reaction	Itching
Eye irritation	Headache

First Aid

Remove victim from source of poison.
Flush affected area with large amounts of water.
Remove clothes affected with poison.
Care for shock.
Monitor breathing.

101. SIGNALS OF AND CARE FOR BITES AND STINGS

INSECT BITES

Signals

Presence of stinger
Pain
Swelling
Possible allergic reaction

Care

Remove stinger.
Wash wound.
Cover.
Apply a cold pack.
Watch for signs of an allergic reaction.

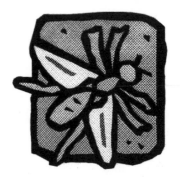

SPIDER BITE/SCORPION STING

Signals

Bite mark
Swelling
Pain
Nausea and vomiting
Difficulty breathing or swallowing

Care

Wash wound.
Apply a cold pack.
Get medical care to receive antivenin.
Call for emergency assistance.

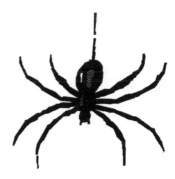

MARINE LIFE STINGS

Signals

Possible marks
Pain
Swelling
Possible allergic reaction

Care

Jellyfish—soak in vinegar.
Stingray—soak area in hot water, clean, and bandage.
Call emergency number for assistance.

SNAKE BITES

Signals

Bite mark
Pain

Care

Wash wound.
Keep bitten part still and lower than the heart.
Call local emergency number.

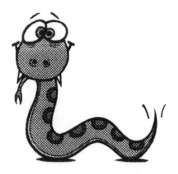

ANIMAL BITES

Signals

Bite mark
Bleeding

Care

Wash area if bleeding is minor.
Control bleeding.
Apply antibiotic ointment.
Cover.
Get medical attention if wound bleeds severely or if you suspect animal has rabies.
Call local emergency number or contact animal control personnel.

Source: American Red Cross Staff, *American Red Cross Community First Aid & Safety*. St. Louis, MO: Mosby-Yearbook, Inc., 1993.

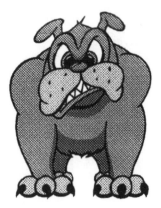

102. SIGNALS OF AND CARE FOR SUDDEN ILLNESS

The American Red Cross states that when a person becomes suddenly ill, he or she often looks and feels sick.

SIGNALS OF SUDDEN ILLNESS

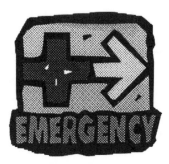

- Feeling lightheaded
- Feeling weak or dizzy
- Feeling confused
- Pale or flushed skin
- Nausea or vomiting
- Difficulty breathing
- Persistent pressure or pain
- Diarrhea
- Seizures
- Inability to move
- Slurred speech
- Difficulty seeing
- Severe headache

CARE FOR SUDDEN ILLNESS

- Help the victim rest comfortably
- Keep the victim from getting chilled or overheated
- Reassure the victim
- Watch for changes in consciousness
- Do not give the victim food or drink unless he or she is fully conscious

103. SIGNALS OF AND CARE FOR DIABETIC EMERGENCIES

SIGNALS OF DIABETIC EMERGENCY

- Dizziness
- Drowsiness
- Confusion
- Rapid breathing
- Rapid pulse
- Felling and looking ill

CARE FOR DIABETIC EMERGENCY

- Check for medic alert tag
- Administer sugar to conscious victim. (Most candy, fruit juices, and nondiet soft drinks contain sufficient sugar to be effective.)
- Do not give unconscious victim anything to eat or drink
- Maintain normal body temperature
- Call emergency medical services (EMS)

104. SIGNALS OF AND CARE FOR STROKE

SIGNALS OF STROKE

➡ Sudden weakness   ➡ Confusion

➡ Difficulty speaking   ➡ Severe headache

➡ Blurred vision   ➡ Ringing in the ears

➡ Pupils of unequal size   ➡ Mood changes

➡ Dizziness   ➡ Unconsciousness

➡ Numbness of face, arm, or leg
   (often on one side of the body)

CARE FOR STROKE

Conscious Victim

Phone EMS.

Have victim rest in comfortable position.

Do not administer food or drink.

Reassure victim.

Place victim on side if vomiting or drooling.

Unconscious Victim

Phone EMS.

Maintain open airway.

Place victim on side to allow fluids to drain from mouth.

Do not leave victim unattended.

105. CAUSES OF AND CARE FOR SEIZURES

CAUSES OF SEIZURES

➡ Head injury   ➡ Infection

➡ Disease   ➡ Epilepsy

➡ Fever

CARE FOR SEIZURES

➡ Do not hold or restrain victim

➡ Do not put anything in the victim's mouth

➡ Protect the victim from injury

➡ Maintain an open airway

➡ Roll victim on side if vomiting occurs

➡ Reassure the victim

➡ Do not leave victim unattended

➡ Call EMS in any of the following situations:

     Seizures last longer than a few minutes
     Victim has repeated seizures
     Injuries are involved
     The cause of the seizure is unknown
     The victim if pregnant
     The victim is diabetic
     The seizure occurs in water
     Victim remains unconscious after the seizure

106. SIGNALS OF AND CARE FOR HEAT-RELATED EMERGENCIES

SIGNALS OF HEAT EMERGENCIES

Heat Exhaustion

Cool, moist, pale, or flushed skin   Nausea or vomiting
Heavy sweating   Exhaustion
Headache   Dizziness
Near normal body temperature

Heat Stroke

Hot, red skin
Rapid, weak pulse
Rapid, shallow breathing
Changes in consciousness
Very high body temperature
Wet skin if the person was sweating from heavy work or exercise; otherwise, dry skin

CARE FOR HEAT EMERGENCIES

Heat Cramps

Get the person to a cooler place and have him or her rest in a comfortable position.
Lightly stretch the affected muscle and replenish fluids.
Give a half glass of cool water every 15 minutes.
Do not give liquids containing alcohol or caffeine.

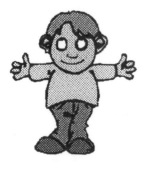

Heat Exhaustion

Get the person out of the heat and into a cooler place.
Remove or loosen tight clothing and apply cool, wet cloth.
Give a half glass of cool water every 15 minutes.
Make sure the person drinks slowly.
Do not give liquids that contain alcohol or caffeine.
Let the victim rest in a comfortable position.
Watch carefully for changes in his or her condition.

Heat Stroke

Heat stroke is a life-threatening situation.
Call local emergency number immediately.
Move the person to a cooler place.
Immerse victim in a cool bath, or wrap wet sheets around the body and fan it.
Watch for signals of breathing problems.
Keep the person lying down, and continue to cool the body any way possible.
If the victim refuses water or is vomiting, or there are changes in the level of consciousness, do not give anything to eat or drink.

107. SIGNALS OF AND CARE FOR COLD-RELATED EMERGENCIES

SIGNALS OF FROSTBITE

➡ There is no feeling in the affected area

➡ Skin appears waxy

➡ Skin is cold to the touch

➡ Skin is discolored

CARE FOR FROSTBITE

➡ Handle area gently

➡ Do not rub affected area

➡ Soak affected area in warm water

➡ Loosely bandage affected area with a dry sterile dressing

➡ Do not break blisters

➡ Seek medical attention

SIGNALS OF HYPOTHERMIA

➡ Shivering

➡ Numbness

➡ Glassy stare

➡ Apathy

➡ Loss of consciousness

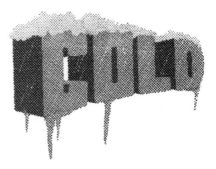

CARE FOR HYPOTHERMIA

➡ Call for emergency medical assistance

➡ Keep victim comfortable

➡ Remove any wet clothing

➡ Dry victim

➡ Warm victim slowly by wrapping in blankets or putting on dry clothing

➡ Move victim to warm, dry area

➡ Apply heat to the victim

➡ Administer warm liquids to conscious victim

➡ Handle victim gently

108. SAFETY TIPS TO PROTECT CHILDREN

➡ Have a plan for dealing with emergencies

➡ Check the environment for fire and burn dangers

➡ Never keep loaded guns where children can reach them

➡ Buckle up children in motor vehicles

➡ Always watch children in or around water

➡ Use gates on stairs

➡ Keep plastic bags, cords, and small objects away from young children

➡ Keep emergency phone numbers, including the poison control number, readily available

➡ Follow safety rules, and teach them to young children

➡ For additional information on children's safety, contact:

CONSUMER PRODUCT SAFETY COMMISSION
Washington, DC 20207
(800) 638-CPSC
Web site: http://www.cpsc.gov

NATIONAL MATERNAL AND CHILD HEALTH CLEARINGHOUSE
8201 Greensboro Drive
Suite 600
McLean, VA 22102
(703) 821-8955
Web site: http://www.circsol.com/mch/
E-mail: nmchc@circsol.com

109. WATER SAFETY PRECAUTIONS

BOATING

➡ Learn proper boating procedures

➡ Use boats that are in good condition

➡ Always wear a life jacket

➡ Observe the load limit of the boat

DIVING

➡ Check water depth before diving

➡ Never dive into unfamiliar water or shallow breaking waves

➡ Never dive from side of diving board

➡ Slide feet first down waterslide

➡ Make sure area is clear before diving

SWIMMING

➡ Follow posted swimming rules

➡ Never swim alone

➡ Swim only when a lifeguard is on duty

➡ Avoid pushing, shoving, and dangerous horseplay

➡ Muscle cramp procedure:

    Do not panic

    Relax

    Float

    Press and squeeze muscle until it relaxes

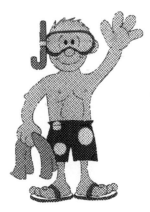

110. SAFETY PRECAUTIONS IN WEATHER-RELATED EMERGENCIES

HURRICANE AND TORNADO

➡ A *watch* means that atmospheric conditions exist for these conditions to develop

➡ A *warning* means that one has been sighted and that instructions will be issued by the National Weather Service

➡ *Hurricane*

   Secure your property

   Go to a shelter, or evacuate the area

➡ *Tornado*

   Go to basement or storm caller

   Go to hallway or bathtub away from windows

   Outside—lie face down in ditch and cover yourself

EARTHQUAKE

➡ If you are inside a building when tremors begin, follow these basic safety procedures:

   Stay in building

   Go to safe spot near where you are standing, such as under a heavy desk

   Go to corner of the room away from anything that may collapse

➡ If you are outdoors when tremors begin, stay away from buildings, trees, and power lines

BLIZZARD

➡ If you are caught outside:

   Keep mouth and nose covered

   Keep moving so that you do not freeze

   Follow a road or fence to the nearest safe area

➡ If you must go outside:

   Wear adequate protection, such as:

   – thermal, woolen undergarments

   – outer garments that repel wind and moisture

   – head, face, and ear coverings

   – extra socks

   – warm boots

   – wool-lined mittens

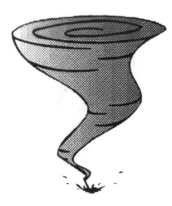

111. SUPPLIES IN A FIRST-AID KIT

The American Red Cross recommends that the following items be stocked in the basic first-aid kit:

- Gauze Pads and Roller Gauze (assorted sizes)
- Adhesive Tape
- Cold Pack
- Plastic Bags
- Disposable Gloves
- Band-Aids (assorted sizes)
- Hand Cleaner
- Small Flashlight and Extra Batteries
- Scissors and Tweezers
- Blanket
- Triangular Bandage
- Syrup of Ipecac
- Antiseptic Ointment
- Activated Charcoal
- First-Aid Manual

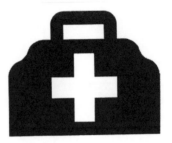

DISEASES AND DISORDERS

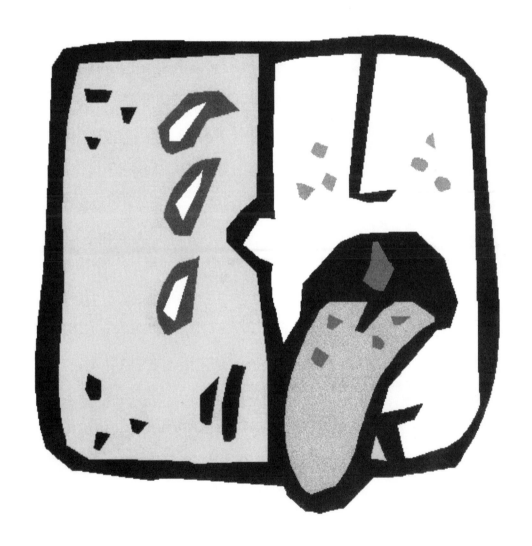

112. COMMON COMMUNICABLE DISEASES

ANTHRAX
Bacterial disease that can infect all warm-blooded animals including man.

BOTULISM
Food poisoning caused by bacterium *Clostridium botulinum*.

CHICKENPOX
Highly communicable disease caused by a member of the herpes virus family.

CHOLERA
Bacterial disease that affects the intestinal tract, caused by a germ called *Vibro cholera*. Six worldwide outbreaks were documented between 1817 and 1911 that resulted in hundreds of thousands of deaths. Currently, only a few cases are recognized in the United States each year.

DIPHTHERIA
An acute bacterial disease that usually affects the tonsils, throat, nose, or skin.

E. COLI
Bacteria that normally live in the intestines of humans and animals. Although most strains of this bacterium are harmless, one particular strain known as E. coli 0157:H7 infection is known to produce a toxin that can cause serious illness.

GONORRHEA
Infection that is spread through sexual contact with another person. Germs are found in the mucous area of the body (the vagina, penis, throat, and rectum).

HAEMOPHILUS INFLUENZA TYPE B (HIB)
One of the most important causes of serious bacterial infection in young children. Hib may cause a variety of diseases such as meningitis (inflammation of the coverings of the spinal cord and brain), blood stream infections, pneumonia, arthritis, and infections of other parts of the body.

HEPATITIS A (INFECTIOUS HEPATITIS)
Common liver disease caused by a specific virus.

HEPATITIS B (SERUM HEPATITIS)
Common liver disease caused by a virus.

HEPATITIS C (NON-A, NON-B HEPATITIS)
Liver disease caused by a recently identified blood-borne virus. Other types of viral hepatitis include hepatitis A (infectious hepatitis), hepatitis B (serum hepatitis), hepatitis D (delta hepatitis), and hepatitis E (a virus transmitted through the feces of an infected person).

HERPES II
Sexually transmitted viral infection characterized by painful sores, usually in the genital area. Once infected, an individual may carry the virus and be subject to recurrent bouts of infection.

INFECTIOUS MONONUCLEOSIS

Viral disease that affects certain blood cells. It is caused by the Epstein-Barr virus (EBV), which is a member of the herpes virus family. Often referred to as "mono." When it strikes young children, the illness is usually so mild that it passes as a common cold or the flu. When it occurs during adolescence or adulthood, however, the disease can be much more serious.

INFLUENZA or FLU

Viral infection of the nose, throat, bronchial tubes, and lungs. The two main types of virus are A and B.

LEPROSY

Rare chronic bacterial disease of the skin, nerves in the hands and feet, and, in some cases, the lining of the nose.

LYME DISEASE

Bacterial infection transmitted by a certain type of tick. May cause symptoms affecting the skin, nervous system, heart and/or joints of an individual.

MALARIA

Mosquito-borne disease caused by any one of four different blood parasites, and a leading cause of debilitating illness.

MEASLES

Acute, highly contagious viral disease capable of producing epidemics common in winter and spring.

MENINGOCOCCAL MENINGITIS

Rare but severe bacterial infection of the bloodstream and meninges (thin lining covering the brain and spinal cord).

MUMPS

Acute viral disease characterized by fever, swelling, and tenderness of one or more of the salivary glands.

NONGONOCOCCAL URETHRITIS (NGV)

Infection of the urethra (the tube running from the bladder through the penis in men or the labia in women through which urine passes) caused by some agent other than gonorrhea. This infection can be caused by any of several different organisms, although the most frequent cause of NGU is a bacterium called *Chlamydia trachomatis* and is a sexually transmitted disease (STD).

PEDICULOSIS (HEAD LICE, BODY LICE, PUBIC LICE, COOTIES, CRABS)

Infestation of the hairy parts of the body or clothing with eggs, larvae, or adults of lice. The crawling stages of this insect feed on human blood, which can result in severe itching. Head lice are usually located on the scalp, crab lice in the pubic area, and body lice along seams of clothing, traveling to the skin to feed.

PERTUSSIS (WHOOPING COUGH)

Highly contagious disease involving the respiratory tract. It is caused by a bacterium that is found in the mouth, nose, and throat of an infected person.

BUBONIC PLAGUE

Rare but severe disease caused by an infection with a type of bacteria that is found in rodents and transmitted to man by fleas.

POLIOMYELITIS (INFANTILE PARALYSIS, POLIO)

Rare viral disease that may affect the central nervous system.

RABIES (HYDROPHOBIA)	Deadly disease caused by a virus present in saliva and the nervous tissue of rabid animals, attacks the nervous system.
RINGWORM	Skin infection caused by a fungus that can affect the scalp, skin, fingers, toe nails, or foot.
ROCKY MOUNTAIN FEVER (TICK-BORNE TYPHUS FEVER) (RMSF)	Disease caused by a rickettsial organism transmitted to humans by the bite of an infected tick.
RUBELLA (GERMAN MEASLES)	Viral disease characterized by fever, rash, and swollen glands.
SALMONELLOSIS	Bacterial infection that affects the intestinal tract and the bloodstream.
SCABIES	Infectious disease of the skin caused by a mite that burrows into the skin.
SHINGLES (HERPES ZOSTER)	Localized, painful infection occurring only in people who have had chickenpox.
SYPHILIS	Bacterial infection, primarily a sexually transmitted disease (STD).
TETANUS (LOCKJAW)	Bacterial disease that affects the nervous system. Due to widespread immunization, tetanus is now a rare disease.
TRICHINOSIS	Food-borne disease caused by a microscopic parasite.
TUBERCULOSIS (TB)	Bacterial disease, usually affecting the lungs (pulmonary TB). Other parts of the body can also be affected, for example, lymph nodes, kidneys, bones, or joints (extrapulmonary TB).
TYPHIOD FEVER	Rare bacterial infection of the intestinal tract and occasionally the bloodstream.
VENEREAL WARTS (GENITAL WARTS)	Common sexually transmitted disease (STD) caused by a specific virus that affects the skin or mucous membranes. The virus usually causes cauliflower-like fleshy growths in moist areas in and around the sex organs.
VIRAL MENINGITIS (NONBACTERIAL MENINGITIS)	Infection of the meninges (a thin lining covering the brain and spinal cord) by any one of a number of different viruses.
YELLOW FEVER (JUNGLE YELLOW FEVER, URBAN YELLOW FEVER)	Mosquito-borne viral disease occurring in tropical and subtropical areas.

113. TYPES OF PATHOGENS AND WAYS THEY CAN BE SPREAD

TYPES OF PATHOGENS

Pathogens are tiny organisms that attack the body's cells and tissues and cause many common diseases.

BACTERIA	One-celled microscopic organism that may cause the spread of infection.
FUNGI	Parasitic living organisms that may cause infections such as ringworm and athlete's foot.
PROTOZOANS	Single-celled organisms that cause diseases such as malaria.
RICKETTSIAS	Bacterialike organisms carried by bloodsucking insects such as ticks to humans; responsible for typhus fever and Rocky Mountain spotted fever.
VIRUS	Small parasitic particle that can attach itself to a cell and cause it to produce identical viruses such as smallpox, chicken pox, and warts.
WORMS	Roundworms and flatworms; can invade the blood and cause such diseases as trichinosis.

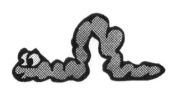

WAYS PATHOGENS CAN BE SPREAD

INDIRECT CONTACT	When an infected person coughs and sneezes, and when an uninfected person touches objects that an infected person has used.
DIRECT CONTACT	When an uninfected person comes into direct physical contact with an infected area on another person.
CONTACT WITH ANIMALS OR INSECTS	When an animal or insect bites a human—can pass the pathogens into the human's body.

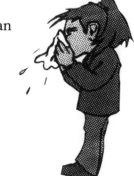

114. TYPES OF VACCINES

Vaccines are usually prepared from dead or weakened viruses and provide immunity to certain diseases by stimulating the production of antibodies against a particular pathogen in the body.

LIVE-VIRUS VACCINE   Weakened live virus that stimulates the production of antibodies in the body, such as those for measles, rubella, and polio.

KILLED-VIRUS VACCINE   Dead virus that stimulates the production of antibodies in the body; weaker than the live-virus vaccine; requires booster shots.

TOXOIDS   Treated toxins that stimulate the production of antibodies in the body, such as those for diphtheria and tetanus.

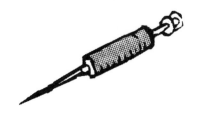

115. RECOMMENDED SCHEDULE FOR ACTIVE IMMUNIZATION

The following is a recommended immunization schedule from the Centers for Disease Control and Prevention:

Birth to 2 Months	Hepatitis B (Hep B)
2 Months	Diphtheria, tetanus, pertussis (DTP), Haemophilus influenza type b (Hib), Polio (OPV)
2 to 4 Months	Hep B
4 Months	DTP, Hib, OPV
6 Months	DTP, Hib
6 to 18 Months	Hep B, OPV
12 to 15 Months	Hib, measles, mumps, rubella, (MMR)
12 to 18 Months	DTP, (DTaP, a slightly different formula of the same vaccine, can be substituted for DTP after 15 months), varicella zoster virus vaccine for chickenpox (VZV)
4 to 6 Years	DTP or DTaP, OPV
4 to 6 Years or 11 to 12 Years	MMR
11 to 12 Years	Hep B, VZV (catch up vaccination)
11 to 16 Years	Tetanus, diphtheria (Td)—should be continued every 10 years thereafter

116. COMMON EXAMPLES OF BIOFEEDBACK

Biofeedback is the process of becoming aware of physical events in your body that are involuntary in order to reestablish normal body conditions. Biofeedback is also used clinically to manage stress, and to relieve migraine and tension headaches, and anxiety disorders.

COMMON EXAMPLES OF BIOFEEDBACK

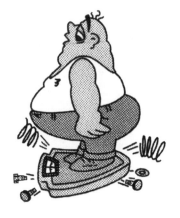

➥ Weighing yourself
➥ Taking your pulse when exercising
➥ Taking your temperature when you are sick
➥ Using instruments to regulate physical processes, such as:
> muscle tension
> brain waves
> skin temperature
> skin resistance

117. SYMPTOMS OF LYME DISEASE

EARLY INFECTION

➥ Brief episodes of joint pain swelling
➥ Facial paralysis (Bell's palsy)
➥ Fever
➥ Headache
➥ Meningitis
➥ Muscle and joint aches
➥ Rash
➥ Stiff Neck
➥ Significant fatigue

> *Less Common:*
> Eye problems such as conjunctivitis
> Heart abnormalities such as heart block and myocarditis

LATE INFECTION

➥ Arthritis, intermittent or chronic

> *Less Common:*
> Neurologic conditions such as encephalitis or confusion
> Skin disorders

118. STEPS TO PREVENT LYME DISEASE

The Centers for Disease Control (CDC) recommends the following:

➡ Avoid tick-infested areas, especially in May, June, and July

➡ Wear light-colored clothing in order to detect ticks easily

➡ Wear long-sleeved shirts and hats

➡ Wear closed shoes with socks

➡ Tuck pant legs into socks or boots

➡ Tuck shirt into pants

➡ Apply insect repellent to clothes and exposed skin (other than face)

➡ Walk in the center of trails

➡ Avoid overgrown grass and brush

➡ Check pets regularly for ticks

➡ After being in tick-infested areas:
Remove, wash, and dry clothing
Inspect the body thoroughly for ticks
Treat tick bites with antibiotics

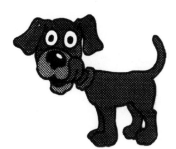

119. SYMPTOMS OF MONONUCLEOSIS

SYMPTOMS

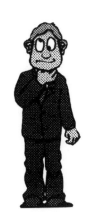

Early symptoms resemble those of the flu:
Severe fatigue
Headache
Sore throat, sometimes very severe
Chills, followed by a fever
Muscle aches

The following additional symptoms may occur:
Swollen lymph nodes, especially in the neck, armpits, or groin
Jaundice (a yellow tinge to the skin and eyes)
A measles-like skin rash anywhere on the face or body; sometimes the rash develops suddenly after taking amoxicillin for a severe sore throat
Bruiselike areas inside the mouth
Soreness in the upper left abdomen (from an enlarged spleen)

120. SYMPTOMS OF HEPATITIS

➡ Fatigue

➡ Mild fever

➡ Muscle or joint aches

➡ Nausea and vomiting

➡ Abdominal pain

➡ Diarrhea or constipation

➡ Loss of appetite

➡ Weakness

➡ Red palms

➡ Lack of nutrition

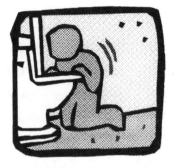

LESS COMMON SYMPTOMS INCLUDE

➡ Dark urine

➡ Light-colored stools

➡ Jaundice

➡ Generalized itching

➡ Altered mental state, stupor, or coma

121. COMMON WAYS HEPATITIS CAN BE SPREAD

HEPATITIS A

➡ Improper handling of food
➡ Contact with household members
➡ Sharing toys at day-care centers
➡ Eating raw shellfish taken from polluted waters

HEPATITIS B

➡ From mother to child at birth
➡ Through sexual contact
➡ Through blood transfusions
➡ Through needle sharing by intravenous drug users

HEPATITIS C

➡ Through contact with blood or contaminated needles
➡ Through blood transfusions

HEPATITIS D

➡ Transmitted from mother to child
➡ Through sexual contact

HEPATITIS E

➡ Through fecal contamination

ALCOHOLIC, TOXIC, AND DRUG-RELATED HEPATITIS

➡ Excessive and chronic consumption of alcohol
➡ Ingestion of environmental toxins
➡ Misuse of certain prescription drugs and over-the-counter medications such as acetaminophen

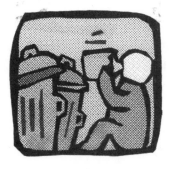

122. THREE BASIC DEFENSES AGAINST INFECTION

SKIN AND MUCOUS MEMBRANES

⟹ Skin

⟹ Mucous membranes

⟹ Cilia and other body hairs (eyelashes)

⟹ Digestive fluids

⟹ Vaginal fluids

⟹ Bacteria-killing secretions
Perspiration
Tears
Saliva
Skin oils

⟹ Reflexes
Coughing
Blinking
Vomiting

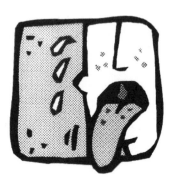

INFLAMMATORY RESPONSES

⟹ Phagocytes (white blood cells)—engulf bacteria and foreign particles and destroy them

⟹ Fever—most pathogens cannot survive in above-normal body temperatures

IMMUNITY

⟹ Lymphocytes (white blood cells)—increase the number of plasma cells, which produce antibodies that attack and destroy foreign cells

⟹ Antibodies—produced by the body in response to invading antigens; can inactivate them

123. GUIDELINES TO REDUCE THE SPREAD OF INFECTION

⟹ Bathe or shower every day to keep your skin, hair, and nails clean

⟹ Avoid sharing eating or drinking utensils

⟹ Store and prepare food in a safe way to prevent food poisoning

⟹ Wash your hands after using the bathroom, after changing diapers, and before preparing or serving food

⟹ If you know you are sick, avoid giving your illness to someone else

⟹ If you are well, avoid contact with people who are sick

124. COMMON ANTIBIOTICS AND METHODS OF ADMINISTRATION

Infectious diseases are treated by antibiotics that harm the bacteria, either by killing them or by preventing them from multiplying.

Common Antibiotics	Methods of Administration
Amoxicillin	Injection
Azithromycin	Orally
Clarithromycin	Topically
Erythromycin	
Neosporin	
Penicillin	

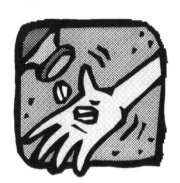

125. COMMON DISEASES AND DISORDERS OF THE MAJOR BODY SYSTEMS

CARDIOVASCULAR SYSTEM

ANEMIA   Red blood cell deficiency.

CONGENITAL HEART DISEASE   Heart defect present at birth.

HEMOPHILIA   Deficiency of certain blood components necessary for rapid blood clotting.

HEART MURMUR   Abnormal heart sound commonly caused by a defective valve.

LEUKEMIA   Cancer of the blood resulting from abnormal white blood cell production.

SICKLE CELL ANEMIA Severe anemia caused by defective hemoglobin in the red blood cells.

DIGESTIVE SYSTEM

APPENDICITIS   Inflammation of the appendix.

CROHN'S DISEASE	Chronic disease of the digestive tract.
GALLSTONES	Small bile crystals that block the bile duct between the gallbladder and the duodenum.
GASTRITIS	Inflammation of the mucous membrane lining the stomach.
HEPATITIS	Inflammation of the liver commonly caused by a viral infection.
HIATAL HERNIA	Condition resulting when the upper part of the stomach pushes through the diaphragm.
PEPTIC ULCER	Open sore in the stomach or duodenum resulting from overproduction of gastric acid.

ENDOCRINE SYSTEM

ADDISON'S DISEASE	Disease resulting from underproductive adrenal glands.
CRETINISM	Condition resulting from a lack of thyroid hormones during the growth years.
CUSHING'S DISEASE	Disease resulting from overproductive adrenal glands.
DIABETES MELLITUS	Condition resulting from the lack of insulin production in the pancreas.

LYMPHATIC SYSTEM

HODGKIN'S DISEASE	Cancer of lymph tissue.
TONSILLITIS	Inflammation of the tonsils.

MUSCULAR SYSTEM

MUSCULAR DYSTROPHY	Genetic disease characterized by a progressive deterioration of the skeletal muscles.
MYASTHENIA GRAVIS	Disease characterized by weak or easily fatigued muscles.

NERVOUS SYSTEM

ALZHEIMER'S DISEASE	Progressive, degenerative disorder resulting in general mental deterioration.
CEREBRAL PALSY	Any of several neurological disorders resulting from brain damage during the developmental stages.
DOWN SYNDROME	Chromosomal abnormality characterized by mild to severe mental retardation.
ENCEPHALITIS	Inflammation of the brain caused by a virus or bacteria.
EPILEPSY	Condition resulting from a sudden surge of nerve impulses in the brain, which can cause seizures.

MENINGITIS	Inflammation of the meninges (membranes around brain and spinal cord) caused by bacteria or a virus.
MULTIPLE SCLEROSIS	Progressive deterioration of the myelin sheath surrounding the nerve fibers.
PARKINSON'S DISEASE	Progressive disease that interferes with the transmission of nerve impulses from motor areas of the brain.
PHENYLKETONURIA (PKU)	Genetic disease causing progressive mental retardation—characterized by the body's inability to break down phenylalanine (an essential amino acid).
POLIOMYELITIS	Viral infection that affects motor neurons in the brain stem and spinal cord.
RABIES	Viral infection of the brain and spinal cord caused by a bite from an infected animal.

SKELETAL SYSTEM

ARTHRITIS	Inflammation and swelling of the joints.
BURSITIS	Inflammation of the bursa (fluid-containing sac) in the joint.
FRACTURE	Any type of break in the bone.
OSTEOMYELITIS	Inflammation of the soft inner surface of the bone.
OSTEOPOROSIS	Disorder resulting from loss of calcium in the bone.
SCOLIOSIS	Lateral curvature of the spine.

RESPIRATORY SYSTEM

BRONCHIAL ASTHMA	Bronchial constriction due to a sensitivity to an allergen.
BRONCHITIS	Inflammation of the lining of the bronchial tubes.
EMPHYSEMA	Destruction of the alveoli due to long-term respiration of foreign particles.
PLEURISY	Inflammation of the lining of the lungs.
PNEUMONIA	Infection of the lungs caused by a virus or bacteria.
TUBERCULOSIS	Infectious bacterial disease involving the growth of tubules on the lungs.

URINARY SYSTEM

CYSTITIS	Bacterial infection of the bladder.
INCONTINENCE	Inability of the body to control the bladder.
KIDNEY STONES	Crystals that form in the kidneys from mineral salts and urea.
URETHRITIS	Inflammation of the urethra.

126. RISK FACTORS FOR HEART DISEASE

➠ Hypertension or high blood pressure (over 140/90).

➠ High cholesterol levels—contribute to the formation of fatty deposits in arteries and increase the chance of a heart attack.

➠ Smoking—decreases the blood's oxygen-carrying capacity and causes the heart to work harder. Smoking also narrows the vessels supplying blood to the arms and legs. The chemicals in cigarette smoke promote the formation of blood clots.

➠ Obesity—when weight is more than 30 percent over the desirable level, a person's chances of developing high blood pressure, high cholesterol, and diabetes increase greatly

➠ Diabetes—increased heart disease risk in people with diabetes who tend to be over-weight and physically inactive, and who have high cholesterol and high blood pressure

➠ Physical inactivity—exercising burns calories, helps control cholesterol, and strengthens the heart muscle

➠ Stress—most scientists agree that impatient people who have emotional outbursts seem to have a higher risk of heart disease

➠ Gender—men have a higher overall risk than women. The difference disappears after women reach menopause.

➠ Family history—heart disease is more common in people with family members who developed heart disease before the age of 55

127. STEPS TO PREVENT HEART DISEASE

➠ Quit smoking, or if you do not smoke, do not start

➠ Avoid the cigarette smoke of others

➠ Reduce the amount of fat you eat, especially saturated fat

➠ Limit intake of foods that are high in cholesterol

➠ Limit intake of salt (sodium)

➠ Include fiber in your diet

➠ Use alcohol only in moderation

➠ Exercise regularly in moderation

➠ Have regular medical checkups

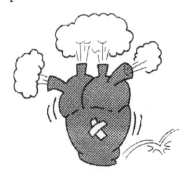

128. TYPES OF CANCER

➠ Anal Cancer
➠ Bladder Cancer
➠ Bone Marrow Cancer
➠ Brain and Spinal Cord Cancer
➠ Breast Cancer
➠ Cervical Cancer
➠ Colorectal Cancer
➠ Endometrial Cancer
➠ Esophageal Cancer
➠ Kidney Cancer (Renal Cell Carcinoma)
➠ Laryngeal Cancer
➠ Liver Cancer
➠ Lung Cancer
➠ Mesothelioma
➠ Non-Hodgkin's Lymphoma
➠ Osteosarcoma Cancer
➠ Ovarian Cancer
➠ Pancreas Cancer
➠ Prostate Cancer
➠ Salivary Gland Cancer
➠ Skin Cancer
➠ Stomach Cancer
➠ Thyroid Cancer
➠ Uterine Cancer

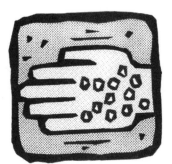

129. WARNING SIGNS OF CANCER

SEVEN CANCER WARNING SIGNS

➠ Change in bowel or bladder habits
➠ A sore that does not heal
➠ Unusual bleeding or discharge
➠ Thickening or lump in breast or elsewhere
➠ Indigestion or difficulty swallowing
➠ Obvious change in wart or mole
➠ Nagging cough or hoarseness

Other warning signs include fatigue and unexplained weight loss.

130.   METHODS OF CANCER TREATMENT

MAJOR TREATMENT APPROACHES

➡ Chemotherapy—a course of treatment using chemicals that destroy cancerous cells
➡ Radiation Therapy—using energy in very high, concentrated doses to destroy cancer cells
➡ Surgery—surgically removing involved cancerous cells, tissue, and organs

OTHER TREATMENT APPROACHES

➡ Alternative treatments
➡ Bone marrow transplantation
➡ Experimental treatments
➡ Hormonal therapy
➡ Hospice
➡ Immunotherapy
➡ Pain management

131.   RISK FACTORS FOR CANCER

The American Cancer Society gives the following as risk factors for cancer:

ALCOHOL

➡ Heavy use of alcohol (especially when accompanied by cigarette smoking or smokeless tobacco use) increases the risk of cancers of the mouth, throat, esophagus, and liver

OCCUPATIONAL HAZARDS

➡ Exposure to nickel, chromate, vinyl chloride, asbestos, and some other industrial chemicals increases the risk of various cancers. Risk from asbestos is greatly increased when combined with cigarette smoking.

RADIATION

➡ Excessive exposure to ionizing radiation (e.g., medical X-rays) can increase cancer risk.

➡ Excessive exposure to radon gas in homes may increase the risk of lung cancer, especially in cigarette smokers. (Check at your local hardware store, or call your local American Cancer Society affiliate about how to order a radon test kit to test your home.)

HORMONE REPLACEMENT THERAPY (HRT)

➡ Hormone replacement therapy after menopause may increase the risk of breast and endometrial cancer. Discuss the pros and cons of these medications with your doctor.

NUTRITION

➡ The risk for breast, colon, gall bladder, prostate, ovarian, and uterine cancers increases if you are overweight

➡ A varied diet that supplies plenty of vegetables and fruits rich in vitamins A and C, and the "cruciferous" vegetables, may reduce the risk of a wide range of cancers

➡ High-fat diets may contribute to the development of cancers of the breast, colon, and prostate

➡ High-fiber foods may help reduce the risk of colon cancer

➡ Salt-cured, smoked, and nitrite-cured foods have been linked to cancer of the esophagus and stomach

SUNLIGHT

➡ Excessive exposure to natural or artificial sunlight increases the cancer risk for the three major kinds of skin cancer (basal cell carcinoma, squamous cell carcinoma, and malignant melanoma)

SMOKING/SMOKELESS TOBACCO

➡ Smoking is responsible for about 1/3 of all cancer deaths

➡ Smokers are at increased risk for cancer of the throat, esophagus, lung, bladder, pancreas, and cervix (women)

➡ The use of chewing tobacco or snuff increases the risk of cancer of the mouth, throat, and esophagus, and is highly habit forming

132. INTERESTING FACTS ABOUT DISEASES AND DISORDERS

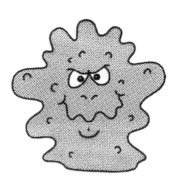

➥ More than 50 million Americans are affected by hypertension (high blood pressure)

➥ Someone died from cardiovascular disease every 33 seconds in the United States in 1995

➥ Of deaths from coronary heart disease, 30%–40% are attributed to obesity and high blood cholesterol

➥ Nicotine hits the brain as a stimulant within 4 seconds after a person has inhaled tobacco, but it then produces an immediate depressant effect

➥ Cigarette smoking is the major single cause of cancer deaths in the United States, causing more deaths than all other drugs combined

➥ Poor dietary and physical activity patterns are associated with 300,000 deaths each year, second only to tobacco

➥ Three ounces of pure alcohol per day, the equivalent of four to six drinks, will put a pregnant woman at high risk for the development of a baby with Fetal Alcohol Syndrome.

➥ The tallest adult on record was 8 feet, 11 inches

➥ The shortest adult on record was 23.2 inches tall

➥ Hyperventilation is produced by a reduced level of carbon dioxide in the blood resulting from excitement or fear

➥ People who spend time outdoors in the winter should avoid the folk remedy for frostnip or frostbite of rubbing snow on the extremity; rubbing can do more damage to the injury

➥ Eating snow when snowbound outdoors for a prolonged period will hasten the freezing process to the body

➥ Hiccups are the result of the diaphragm suddenly contracting

➥ The record holder for the longest case of hiccups was a man in Iowa who hiccupped for over 64 years

➥ "Anthrax," the Greek word for "coal," is so named because a sign of skin anthrax is a carbuncle or cluster of boils that appear as a hard black center surrounded with bright red inflammation

➥ Although Anthrax is not generally a human disease but an infection of animals, humans can get it. Nearly 60,000 people in southern Europe died of anthrax in 1613, and it has been recognized in America since Colonial days.

➥ About 16 million Americans have diabetes. It is the leading cause of new cases of blindness and lower extremity amputations.

➥ The leading cause of physical disability among Americans aged 15 years and older is arthritis or rheumatism; the second cause is back or spine problems; third, heart trouble.

SEXUALLY TRANSMITTED INFECTIONS, HIV, AND AIDS

133. COMMON SEXUALLY TRANSMITTED INFECTIONS (STI)

- Chancroid
- Chlamydia
- Cytomegalovirus (CMV)
- Genital Warts
- Gonorrhea
- Hepatitis B Virus (HBV)
- Herpes
- Human Immunodeficiency Virus (HIV)
- Human Papilloma Virus (HPV)
- Molluscum Contagiosum
- Pelvic Inflammatory Disease (PID)
- Pediculosis Pubis (Pubic Lice)
- Scabies
- Syphilis
- Trichomoniasis
- Urinary Tract Infections

134. GENERAL SYMPTOMS IN FEMALES

If any of the following symptoms are present in the genital area, it is necessary to see a clinician immediately.

- Abnormal discharges from the vagina
- Odorous discharges from the vagina
- Abnormal discharges from the rectum
- Odorous discharges from the rectum
- Bleeding
- Blisters
- Boils
- Buboes
- Burning sensations
- Cervicitis
- Chancres
- Growths
- Irritations
- Itching
- Menstrual irregularities
- Painful intercourse
- Pains
- Polyps
- Pus
- Rashes
- Sores
- Swelling
- Tenderness
- Ulcers
- Urine changes
- Vaginal yeast infections
- Warts

135. GENERAL SYMPTOMS IN MALES

If any of the following symptoms are present in the genital area, it is necessary to see a clinician immediately.

- Abnormal discharges from the penis
- Odorous discharges from the penis
- Abnormal discharges from the rectum
- Odorous discharges from the rectum
- Bleeding
- Blisters
- Boils
- Buboes
- Burning sensations
- Chancres
- Growths
- Irritations

- Itching
- Painful intercourse
- Pains
- Polyps
- Pus
- Rashes
- Sores
- Swelling
- Tenderness
- Ulcers
- Urine changes
- Warts

136. OTHER SYMPTOMS OF SEXUALLY TRANSMITTED INFECTIONS

Some symptoms of sexually transmitted infections are similar to those of other infections and may not show up in the genital area. Seek medical advice if any of the following symptoms persist:

- Abdominal pain
- Aching joints
- Appetite loss
- Bowel problems
- Chills
- Coatings of the mouth, throat, or vagina
- Coughs
- Diarrhea
- Discolored skin
- Fatigue
- Fevers
- General weakness
- Growths
- Hair loss

- Hearing loss
- Headaches
- Jaundice
- Lightheadedness
- Mental disorders
- Muscular pain
- Nausea
- Night sweats
- Sore throat
- Swollen glands
- Vision loss
- Vomiting
- Weight loss that is constant, rapid, or unexplained

137. MODES OF TRANSMISSION OF SEXUALLY TRANSMITTED INFECTIONS

INFECTION	MODE OF TRANSMISSION
CHANCROID	Vaginal, anal, and oral intercourse.
CHLAMYDIA	Vaginal and anal intercourse. From the birth canal to the fetus. Rarely, from the hand to the eye.

CYTOMEGALOVIRUS	In saliva, blood, cervical and vaginal secretions, urine, and breast milk by:
	    Close personal contact
	    Vaginal, anal, and oral intercourse
	    Blood transfusion
	    Sharing IV drug equipment
	    Pregnancy, childbirth, and breastfeeding.

HUMAN PAPILLOMA VIRUS	Vaginal and anal intercourse. Very rarely, genital warts spread to the fetus during childbirth.
GONORRHEA	Vaginal, anal, and oral intercourse.

HEPATITIS B VIRUS	In semen, saliva, blood, and urine by:
	    Intimate and sexual contact from kissing to vaginal, anal, and oral intercourse
	    Use of unclean needles to inject drugs
	    Accidental sticks with contaminated needles in the course of health care.

HERPES	Touching, sexual intimacy—including kissing. Vaginal, anal, and oral intercourse.

HIV	In blood, semen, vaginal secretions, and breast milk by:
	    Anal and vaginal intercourse—less commonly transmitted through oral sex
	    Sharing contaminated IV drug needles
	    Transfusion of contaminated blood products
	    Childbirth
	    Breastfeeding
	    Accidental sticks with contaminated needles in the course of health care.

MOLLUSCUM CONTAGIOSUM	Vaginal, anal, and oral intercourse. Other intimate contact. Children may become infected through casual contact.
TRICHOMONIASIS	Vaginal intercourse.
SCABIES	Close personal contact. Bedding and clothing.
PUBIC LICE	Contact with infected bedding, clothing, upholstered furniture, and toilet seats. Intimate and sexual contact.
URINARY TRACT INFECTIONS	Sex play that brings fecal material into contact with the vagina and urethra. For some women, the use of a diaphragm. For men, unprotected anal intercourse.

138. RISKY BEHAVIORS KNOWN TO TRANSMIT SEXUALLY TRANSMITTED INFECTIONS

➡ Having sex with an infected person

➡ Having sex with multiple sex partners

➡ Having sex with a partner who has had multiple sex partners

➡ Having sex with a partner who uses intravenous drugs

➡ Intimate contact (including kissing) with a person who has lesions, ulcers, blisters, or sores that contain STI pathogens.

➡ Failing to practice good personal hygiene

➡ Having contact with infected objects, clothing, or bed linens

➡ Sharing an infected IV drug needle or syringe

➡ Failing to take precautions when exposed to infected blood or blood products

➡ Having a blood transfusion with infected blood

➡ Sharing an infected needle when getting a tattoo, having ears pierced, or performing a ceremony to become a blood-brother or blood-sister

Source: Education for Sexuality and HIV/AIDS. Blacklick, OH: Meeks Heit Publishing Company, 1993.

139. STI, HIV, AND AIDS TERMINOLOGY

ABSTINENCE	Choosing not to engage in sexual intercourse.
ACQUIRED IMMUNO-DEFICIENCY SYNDROME (AIDS)	The final stage of HIV infection during which there is a significant decrease in the disease-fighting cells inside the body.
ANTIBODIES	Proteins produced by B cells that help destroy pathogens inside the body.
AZT	A drug commonly used in the treatment of HIV-infected individuals.
B CELLS	The blood cells that produce antibodies.
CHANCRE	A hard, round, painless sore with raised edges resulting from syphilis.
ENZYME-LINKED IMMUNOSORBENT ASSAY (ELISA) TEST	A test that detects antibodies developed by the human immune system in response to the presence of HIV.

HELPER T CELLS	White blood cells that signal B cells to produce antibodies.
HUMAN IMMUNODEFI-CIENCY VIRUS (HIV)	The pathogen that causes AIDS.
KAPOSI'S SARCOMA	A type of cancer that is usually associated with persons who have AIDS.
LYMPHADENOPATHY	The presence of swollen lymph glands throughout the body.
MACROPHAGE	A large cell that acts as a scavenger by engulfing and destroying pathogens.
PNEUMOCYSTIS CARINII PNEU-MONIA	An inflammation of the lungs that is usually associated with AIDS.
SEXUALLY TRANSMITTED INFECTIONS (STI)	Infections caused by pathogens that are transmitted from an infected person to an uninfected person during intimate sexual contact.
VAGINITIS	An irritation or inflammation of the vagina, usually accompanied by a discharge.
WESTERN BLOT TEST	A blood test that is used to confirm the results of a positive ELISA test.

Source: Education for Sexuality and HIV/AIDS. Blacklick, OH: Meeks Heit Publishing Company, 1993.

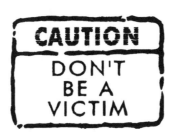

140. HOW THE BODY DEFENDS ITSELF AGAINST ILLNESS

The immune system keeps the body free of infection by constantly fighting pathogens that enter the body. The immune system includes two main types of defenses. One type is nonspecific resistance. Another type is specific resistance. Both types work together to protect the body against pathogens that could cause harm.

NONSPECIFIC RESISTANCE

MECHANICAL MECHANISMS	Skin prevents pathogens from entering the body.
	Mucous membranes in mouth, nose, and bronchial tubes have mucus that traps pathogens.
	Some mucous membranes have cilia (tiny hairs) that trap pathogens, which are then expelled when coughing or sneezing.
	Tears and saliva help carry pathogens away.
CHEMICAL BARRIERS	Chemicals on the surface of tears, sweat, and saliva cells can kill pathogens or prevent them from entering the body.
	Digestive juices of the stomach can destroy some pathogens that may be swallowed with food.
	Other chemicals cause body changes that help cells inside the body to fight pathogens.
CELLS	Phagocytes (certain types of white blood cells) travel through the bloodstream and group together to destroy foreign substances.
INFLAMMATORY RESPONSE	After certain pathogens enter the body, chemicals are released which cause the blood vessels to dilate and allow increased blood flow. The increased blood flow brings phagocytes to the area to leave the blood and enter the tissues. This swelling continues until the pathogens are destroyed.

SPECIFIC RESISTANCE

LYMPHOCYTE	A type of white blood cell that fights pathogens.
ANTIBODIES	Proteins that destroy or neutralize pathogens.

141. RISKY BEHAVIORS KNOWN TO TRANSMIT HIV

HIV is transmitted in blood, semen, breast milk, and vaginal fluids during the following risky behaviors:

➡ Unprotected sex with a person who has HIV

➡ Sharing needles or syringes with someone who has HIV

➡ Receiving a transfusion of infected blood or blood products

➡ Getting HIV-infected blood, semen, or vaginal secretions into open wounds or sores

➡ Receiving tissue or organs transplanted from a donor with HIV

➡ Becoming artificially inseminated with the sperm of a man who has HIV

➡ Becoming accidentally punctured or cut with a needle or surgical instrument contaminated with HIV

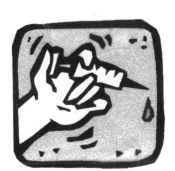

The virus may pass from an infected woman to the fetus during pregnancy or childbirth.

Breastfeeding may pass the virus to an infant.

Source: Planned Parenthood Federation of America.

142. HOW HIV IS *NOT* TRANSMITTED

The transmission of HIV will not occur if risk situations and risk behaviors are avoided.

HIV IS NOT TRANSMITTED BY:

➡ Hugging

➡ Shaking hands

➡ Mosquitoes or other insects

➡ Coughing

➡ Sneezing

➡ Sharing bathroom facilities

➡ Donating blood

➡ Sharing towels

➡ Sharing eating utensils

➡ Sharing a comb or brush

➡ Any other casual contact

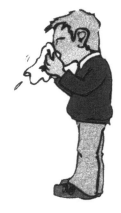

143. HOW HIV INFECTION CAN BE PREVENTED

➠ Knowledge—learn about the disease and apply that knowledge

➠ Abstain from oral, anal, and vaginal intercourse

➠ If you choose to have sexual intercourse:
  Consider your partner's HIV status. Both you and your partner should be tested.
  Have safer sex to reduce the risk of exchanging blood, semen, or vaginal secretions with your partner.
  Use a latex condom from start to finish every time you have vaginal or anal intercourse.

➠ Do not use illegal IV drugs

➠ Do not share needles or syringes

➠ Do not share items that may have blood on them such as, razors, toothbrushes, needles for tattooing, and blades for ritual cutting and scarring

➠ Do not make sexual decisions under the influence of alcohol or other drugs

➠ Be tested for sexually transmitted infections every year. Women and men with open sores from herpes, syphilis, or chancroid are more susceptible to HIV.

Adapted from: AIDS & HIV: Questions & Answers, Planned Parenthood Federation of America.

144. SYMPTOMS OF HIV DISEASE AND AIDS

SYMPTOMS INCLUDE:

➠ A thick, whitish coating of the tongue or mouth (thrush) that is caused by a yeast infection and sometimes accompanied by a sore throat

➠ Severe or recurring vaginal yeast infections

➠ Chronic Pelvic Inflammatory Disease (PID)

➠ Periods of extreme and unexplained fatigue that may be combined with headaches, lightheadedness, and/or dizziness

➠ Rapid loss of more than 10 pounds of weight that is not due to increased physical exercise or dieting

➠ Bruising more easily than normal

➠ Long-lasting occurrences of diarrhea

➠ Recurring fevers and/or night sweats

➠ Swelling or hardening of glands located in the throat, armpit, or groin

➠ Periods of continued, deep, dry coughing

➠ Increasing shortness of breath

➠ The appearance of discolored or purplish growths on the skin or inside the mouth

➠ Unexplained bleeding from growths on the skin, from mucus membranes, or from any opening in the body

➠ Recurring or unusual skin rashes

➠ Severe numbness or pain in the hands or feet, the loss of muscle control and reflex, paralysis or loss of muscle strength

➠ An altered state of consciousness, personality change, or mental deterioration

Such symptoms are often unrelated to HIV disease. Often, when symptoms of HIV disease appear in women, they are often mistaken for those of less serious conditions. Consult your clinician if any of these symptoms persist.

Source: AIDS & HIV: Questions & Answers, Planned Parenthood Federation of America.

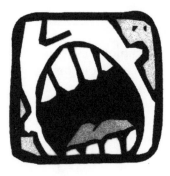

© 1999 by The Center for Applied Research in Education

145. HIV DIAGNOSTIC TESTS

When a pathogen enters the body, the immune system produces antibodies to fight and destroy the pathogen. Although the immune system does produce antibodies to fight HIV, these antibodies are not effective in preventing HIV infection. Finding these antibodies in the blood indicate that a person is infected with HIV. The following tests are used to detect the presence of HIV antibodies in the bloodstream:

TYPE OF TEST

ELISA (Enzyme-Linked Immunosorbent Assay)

One ELISA is given. If the person tests positive, two more tests are done. If, after three tests, two or three are positive, then the Western Blot test is done to confirm the results.

Western Blot Test

This is a more expensive test but is very specific in identifying HIV antibodies.

TEST RESULTS

Positive Result

The person has HIV antibodies in his or her bloodstream.

Negative Result

There are no HIV antibodies in the sample of blood. This does not mean that the person is uninfected because it may take the body from two weeks to six months or longer to develop HIV antibodies. It is best to be retested in six months.

The following are tests that are done after a person is known to have HIV:

TYPE OF TEST

Complete Blood Count

A standard test that measures and analyzes the different types of cells that make up the blood including:

White Blood Cells (WBC)

Measures the number of white blood cells in a cubic millimeter of blood (about one teaspoon). The normal count ranges from 4,000 to 11,000 per cubic millimeter in an average healthy adult.

Red Blood Cells (RBC)

Measures the number of red blood cells in a cubic millimeter of blood. Normal ranges for men are from 4.5–6.1, and for women are 4.0–5.3.

Platelets

These are a part of the blood that is necessary for clotting. Normal count is between 150,000 and 440,000.

Hemoglobin

A protein in RBCs that carries oxygen to the body. Normal levels are 12.0–16.0 grams per deciliter in women and 14.0–18.0 grams per deciliter in men.

Hematocrit

The volume of RBCs in the blood expressed as a percentage of total blood volume. Normal ranges are 40–54% in men and 37–47% in women.

Three Red Cell Measures

Mean Corpuscular Volume (MCV)—measures the average size of an individual red blood cell. The average range is 80 – 100 femtoliters.

Mean Corpuscular Hemoglobin (MCH).

Mean Corpuscular Hemoglobin Concentration (MCHC)—MHC and MCHC measure the amount and volume of hemoglobin in the average cell.

White Cell Differential

This is a breakdown of the different types of WBCs as percentages of the total WBC count.

Chemistry Screen

A chemistry panel examines the levels of 25 different chemicals in the blood and can help determine if the body is functioning properly. Some important values are:

Cholesterol and Triglycerides

These are fatty substances in the blood and are used to measure risk for coronary heart disease and nutritional status. Normal cholesterol levels are 150–250 mg/dl. Triglycerides can range from 47–175 mg/dl.

Amylase

An enzyme secreted by the salivary glands in the mouth and the pancreas.

Liver Functioning Tests

These tests help to determine liver status. Examples include:

Alkaline Phosphatase

Bilirubin

Kidney Functioning Tests

These tests help to determine kidney status. Examples include:

Creatinine

BUN (Blood Urea Nitrogen)

Glucose

This is a sugar in the blood. Normal levels are 60–120 milligrams per deciliter.

Proteins

Albumin and globulin are the two major types of protein in the blood.

Lymphocyte Subsets

Monitoring lymphocyte counts is one way to assess immune system deficiency. The three main groups of lymphocytes are:

B Cells

These cells provide antibodies to neutralize bacteria and viruses.

T Cells

The cells themselves, and not antibodies, kill infectious particles and cells. Some examples of T Cells are:

> CD4+
>
> CD8+

Natural Killer Cells

Viral Load Tests

These are new diagnostic tests that can detect and measure HIV RNA in the plasma of almost all HIV-infected individuals. The various tests are appropriate for different stages of HIV disease. The three main types of test are:

Q-PCR (Quantitative Polymerase Chain Reaction)

bDNA (branched-chain DNA)

NASBA (Nucleic Acid Sequence-Based Amplification)

Less Frequent Routine Tests

These are considered routine in HIV-positive individuals, but do not need to be performed as frequently.

PPD Skin Test

This is done to detect prior tuberculosis exposure.

Chest X-Rays

This and a sputum culture is used to determine the presence of active TB disease.

Pap Smears

Women should have this test done every 6–12 months. A sample of tissue is taken from the cervix and the cervical canal to detect abnormal or cancerous cells.

Source: Project Inform, San Francisco, California, 1997.

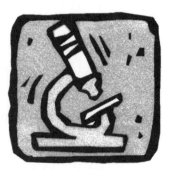

146. HOW AIDS IS DIAGNOSED

Diagnosis of AIDS is based on several factors, including the presence of HIV antibodies and

➠ Blood tests showing that the count of white blood cells, called T lymphocytes, has fallen below 200 per milliliter, or

➠ The presence of one or more opportunistic infections included in the U.S. Centers for Disease Control and Prevention's (CDC) definition of AIDS.

Source: AIDS & HIV: Questions & Answers, Planned Parenthood Federation of America.

147. INFECTIONS INCLUDED IN THE CDC'S DEFINITION OF AIDS

According to the Centers for Disease Control (CDC), AIDS includes a variety of viral, bacterial, fungal, and parasitic infections. It also includes certain cancers. These infections and cancers may affect the digestive, nervous, respiratory, muscular, circulatory, and lymphatic, as well as the immune systems of the body.

The following conditions are also included in the definition of AIDS:

➠ **HIV Wasting Syndrome**—an involuntary loss of 10 percent or more of normal weight. It is often associated with chronic diarrhea or weakness and fever caused by HIV

➠ **HIV Infection of the Brain**—also called AIDS-Dementia, HIV-Dementia, or HIV-Encephalopathy

➠ **Pneumocystis Carinii Pneumonia** and various other forms of pneumonia

➠ **Tuberculosis**

➠ **Kaposi's Sarcoma**, cervical cancer and various other types of cancer

Adapted from: AIDS & HIV: Questions & Answers, Planned Parenthood Federation of America.

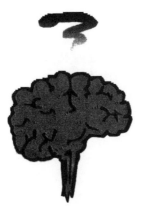

148. MEDICAL TREATMENTS FOR PEOPLE WITH HIV DISEASE

Research has yet to provide one or more definitive treatments for HIV disease. Here are several useful types of intervention that can be taken against HIV, but no one strategy, alone, is sufficient:

GENERAL HEALTH MAINTAINENCE

➡ Proper nutrition
➡ Adequate rest
➡ Avoidance of alcohol, tobacco, other drugs, and unnecessary stress
➡ Exercise and fresh air

SUPPORTIVE THERAPIES

➡ Stress reduction
➡ Massage
➡ Visualization
➡ Yoga and relaxation techniques
➡ Psychological support
➡ Spiritual support

ANTIRETROVIRAL TREATMENTS

These treatments are chemical drugs that interfere with HIV's life cycle or its ability to reproduce. They include:

Reverse Transcriptase Inhibitors

These drugs work by inhibiting an enzyme—reverse transcriptase—which the virus needs to take over a cell's genetic machinery.

Nucleoside Analogs
Examples:
ddI (didanosine, Videx®)
d4T (stavudine, Zerit®)
AZT (also called zidovudine or Retrovir®)
ddC (dideoxycytidine, HIVID®)
3TC (lamivudine, Epivir®)

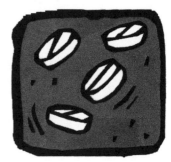

Non-Nucleoside Analogs
Examples:
Nevirapine (Viramune®)
Delavirdine (Rescriptor®)

Protease Inhibitors

These drugs target a different enzyme of the virus—protease—which is essential for HIV to make working copies of itself.

Examples:

Nelfinavir (VIRACEPT®)
Saquinavir (Invirase(TM))
Ritonavir (Novir®)
Indinavir (Crixivan®)

Source: Project Inform, San Francisco, CA, 1997.
National Minority AIDS Council (NMAC), Washington, DC.
AIDS Treatment News, Issue #269, John S. James, April 18, 1997.

Source: Toner, Patricia Rizzo, *Sex Education Activities*. West Nyack, NY: The Center for Applied Research in Education, 1993.

149. SEXUALLY TRANSMITTED INFECTIONS FACT CHART

Disease	Pathogen	Where	How	Symptoms
Vaginitis	chlamydia gardnerella herpes candidiasis herpes trichomonas mycoplasma (agents)	vagina penis anus throat	usually sex but sometimes without sex	pain, discharge, irritation, redness, itching, odor, or asymptomatic
Pubic Lice	pediculosis pubis	pubic hair	sex bedding toilets clothing	itching, rash, pinhead-sized blood spots on underwear
Trichomoniasis	protozoan parasite	vagina	common after menstrua-tion, sex	odorous, yellow discharge, itching, burning while urinating, urethra and bladder infections
Scabies	parasitic mite that burrows under the skin	skin contact	sex, but sometimes no sex	itching in the genital area
Gonorrhea	neisseria gonorrhea bacteria	penis vagina anus throat	direct mucous membrane contact during sex	burning discharge from penis, most women have no symptoms, can cause sterility, arthritis
Genital Warts	human papilloma virus	genitals anus	sex	warts on genitals and anus

Hepatitis	hepatitis A virus	mouth	anal-oral sex, contaminated water	flu-like symptoms, dark urine, abdominal pain, jaundice
		penis vagina anus		
	hepatitis B virus	mouth skin breaks blood	saliva, sex, blood, needles, etc.	
Non-Gonococcal Urethritis (NGU)	chlamydia ureaplasma myco-plasma trichomonas (agents)	penis vagina anus throat	direct mucous membrane contact during sex	men—watery or milky discharge from penis women—burning urination
AIDS	HIV human immuno-deficiency virus	penis, vagina, mouth, rectum, blood, mucous membranes	sex, sharing drug needles, mother to baby, transfusion	skin rashes, diarrhea, fever, weight loss, dry cough, swollen glands, loss of appetite, opportunistic infections, death
Chlamydia	chlamydia trachomatis bacteria	penis, vagina, anus, mouth	sex	painful urination, watery discharge, itching, burning of genitals, pelvic pain, bleeding between periods
Genital Herpes	herpes simplex II virus	penis, vagina, anus, mouth, transfer to eyes if sore is touched	direct, intimate contact	painful blisters or sores on the genitals, swollen glands, fever, headaches, tiredness
Syphilis	treponema pallidum bacteria	penis, vagina, anus, mouth, break in skin	congenital, mucous membrane contact w/ sores during sex	"Chancre" which goes away, fatigue, fever, sores, rash, hair loss, nervous system damage, insanity, death

Source: Toner, Patricia Rizzo, *Sex Education Activities.* West Nyack, NY: The Center for Applied Research in Education, 1993.

Section 8

FAMILY PLANNING

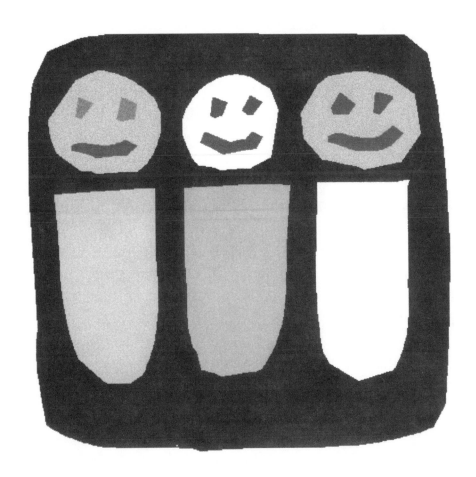

150. CONTRACEPTION THROUGH THE AGES

1800s B.C. A pessary of fermented dough and crocodile dung was mentioned in the Kahun Papyrus, an Egyptian medical manual, as a birth control measure. Because crocodile dung is among the most acidic of animal dung, it may have worked as a spermicide.

1300s B.C. Men in Egypt wore decorative linen covers on their penises. Sheepskin and snakeskin came into fashion in later centuries.

460(?) – 370(?) B.C. Queen Anne's Lace, or Wild Carrot, was mentioned as an oral contraceptive and abortifacient in Hippocrates' writings. Since some sources also record its use for birth control some 2,000 years ago, it may have been in common usage for centuries.

400s B.C. Silphium, another one of the oldest known effective plants for birth control, was used until the 3rd or 4th century A.D. when it became extinct.

200 A.D. Women used spongy substances, much like tampons, as sperm barriers.

MIDDLE AGES, EUROPE Women wore the bones and dried testicles of a weasel or a bone from the right side of a black cat to prevent conception. Another common method was to wear the earwax of a mule as an amulet.

1500s Gabriele Fallopius, for whom Fallopian tubes are named, made a linen cloth to fit over the penis. It was most likely intended to protect against venereal disease rather than as a birth control device.

1880s The invention of the diaphragm marked a new age in birth control.

1920s The "block pessary," a six-sided wooden block, concave on each side, was designed to fit into the vagina with the assumption that one of the concave sides would cover the cervix.

1960 The Food and Drug Administration (FDA) approved the birth control pill for marketing. The pill came as a result of the discovery that progesterone blocks ovulation. The first pills had 10% more progesterone and 20% more estrogen than those currently prescribed.

1971 The Dalkon Shield IUD was first marketed by the A.H. Robins Company.

1973 Landmark Roe v. Wade decision by the Supreme Court legalized abortion in the United States.

1974   A. Albert Yuzpe, a Canadian professor, published the first studies showing that emergency contraceptive pills (ECPs) are effective and safe. The "Yuzpe Regimen," named for him, calls for a dose of estrogen and progestin taken within 72 hours of intercourse, followed by another dose 12 hours later.

1974   The Dalkon Shield was taken off the market in the United States after it was found to have caused pelvic inflammatory disease, spontaneous septic abortions and miscarriages resulting in several deaths.

1983   The sponge received FDA approval as a nonprescription birth control measure.

LATE 1980s   Contraceptive researchers discovered that Queen Anne's lace blocks production of progesterone & inhibits fetal and ovarian growth in mice. It is still a folk medicine method of morning-after contraception, taken by drinking the seeds in a glass of water

1988   The cervical cap was approved for use in the United States, although other versions existed much earlier.

1990   Norplant® received FDA approval.

1992   Depo-Provera® received FDA approval. It endured some 20 years of controversy before it was approved for contraceptive use in the United States.

1993   Reality®, the first female condom, was approved after more than five years of FDA review.

1994   Norma McCorvey, the "Jane Roe" of Roe v. Wade, published her autobiography including details of reform school, drug and alcohol abuse, an abusive husband, a second unwed pregnancy and more. She had confessed sometime during the 80s that her tale of rape in 1970 was a lie; she was an unwed mother who later placed the child for adoption.

1995   Approximately one-third of the 190 million pregnancies in the world in 1995 ended in abortion; the same proportion applied to the United States.

1996   Reproductive Health Technologies Project and Bridging the Gap, Inc. offered a national ECP hotline (1-888-NOT-2-LATE) to give callers ECP information and referrals of clinics and doctors willing to prescribe ECPs.

1998   Sterilization is the most used contraceptive in virtually all the world's regions, including the United States.

1998 (SEPTEMBER) The FDA approved Gynetics, Inc.'s application to market the PRE-VENO Emergency Contraceptive Kit, making it the first commercial ECP product advertised to women in the United States.

151. FACTS ABOUT TEEN SEXUAL BEHAVIOR

➡ Rates of teen sexual behavior have risen throughout the last thirty years

➡ The percentage of eighteen-year-old women who have had intercourse at least once is 56 percent

➡ The percentage of men who have had intercourse by age eighteen is 73 percent

➡ Percent of all adolescents who have participated in:

Kissing	Over 90%
Deep Kissing	79%
Touching "above the waist"	72%
Touching "below the waist"	54%

➡ Percent of teens who are sexually active by age:

12 years old	9%
14 years old	23%
18 years old	71%

➡ In the United States, 25% of the teens who have had sexual intercourse will become infected with a sexually transmitted infection (STI)

➡ The most common STIs in teenagers are gonorrhea, syphilis, and chlamydia

➡ The majority of people who developed AIDS in their twenties were probably infected with HIV in their teens

➡ The U.S. has the highest rate of teenage pregnancy, abortion, and birth in the industrialized world

Source: Thacker, Netha L., and Kathleen R. Miner, *Abstinence: Health Facts*. Santa Cruz, California: ETR Associates, 1996.

152. REASONS WHY TEENS CHOOSE ABSTINENCE

In a 1994 survey, high school students offered the following reasons for choosing abstinence:

- ➡ Want to wait for a committed relationship — 87%
- ➡ Worry about STD — 85%
- ➡ Worry about pregnancy — 84%
- ➡ Want to wait until older — 84%
- ➡ Worry about HIV/AIDS — 83%
- ➡ Waiting to meet the right person — 80%
- ➡ Just not ready for sex — 79%
- ➡ Want to wait until marriage — 71%
- ➡ Against religious beliefs — 40%
- ➡ Lack of opportunity — 38%

Source: Starch, Roper, *Teen Talk About Sex: Adolescent Sexuality in the 90s—A Survey of High School Students.* New York: SIECUS, 1994.

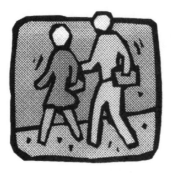

153. NATURAL FAMILY PLANNING METHODS

METHOD	DESCRIPTION
TOTAL ABSTINENCE	No sexual intercourse. EFFECTIVENESS: 100%
CALENDAR CHARTING	Menstrual cycle is charted for eight months in an attempt to predict ovulation. During ovulation, abstinence is practiced. Ovulation is difficult to predict and is affected by illness and stress. EFFECTIVENESS: 70%
BASAL BODY TEMPERATURE (BBT)	Chart BBT daily to detect the higher body temperature during ovulation. Abstain during ovulation. Ovulation is difficult to predict and is affected by illness and stress. EFFECTIVENESS: 75–80%
CERVICAL MUCUS	Observe mucus to detect changes in cervical secretions that occur during ovulation. Abstain during ovulation. It is difficult to detect changes, since other factors affect secretions. EFFECTIVENESS: 75–80%
SYMPTOTHERMAL METHOD	This method employs the use of basal body temperature (BBT) and cervical mucus observation to predict ovulation. Abstain during ovulation. Ovulation is difficult to predict and is affected by illness and stress. EFFECTIVENESS: 75–80%

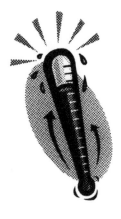

154. BARRIER METHODS OF CONTRACEPTION

METHOD	DESCRIPTION
MALE CONDOM	Rubber or animal skin sheath is placed over the erect penis. This prevents semen from entering the vagina. EFFECTIVENESS: 85% if no human error
FEMALE CONDOM	Also known as the vaginal pouch. A disposable sheath designed to protect the woman from pregnancy and STIs by lining the vagina. EFFECTIVENESS: 79%
CERVICAL CAP	A latex, dome-shaped device that fits snugly over the cervix. This blocks the passage of sperm into the uterus. EFFECTIVENESS: 75%
DIAPHRAGM	A dome-shaped rubber cup with a flexible rim that is used with spermicidal gel. This covers the cervix and blocks the passage of sperm into the uterus. EFFECTIVENESS: 75% if no human error and if used with gel
CONTRACEPTIVE SPONGE	Small, pillow-shaped sponge that contains a spermicide. A concave dimple on one side fits over the cervix and acts as a barrier. The sponge was taken off the market by its manufacturer but may return in the future. EFFECTIVENESS: 75% if no human error

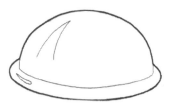

155. CHEMICAL METHODS OF CONTRACEPTION

METHOD	DESCRIPTION
ORAL CONTRA-CEPTIVES (THE PILL)	Tablets of synthetic hormones, which prevent pregnancy by inhibiting the monthly release of the egg from the ovaries. EFFECTIVENESS: 99% if no human error
SPERMICIDES	Chemicals (nonoxynol-9, octoxynol) containing surfactants that destroy the sperm cell membrane. Spermicides can be foam, gel, cream, or suppositories. EFFECTIVENESS: 75% if no human error
VAGINAL CONTRA-CEPTIVE FILM (VCF)	A square of film containing the spermicide, nonoxynol-9. The film is placed high in the vagina against the cervix, where it dissolves at body temperature. EFFECTIVENESS: 75% if no human error
INTRA-UTERINE DEVICE (IUD)	A flexible, usually plastic, device inserted into the uterus by a doctor during menstruation. May contain hormones. The IUD may affect the sperm, egg, fertilization, implantation, or the endometrium to prevent pregnancy. EFFECTIVENESS: 95%
NORPLANT®	Six capsules filled with the hormone leuonorgestrel are implanted into the upper arm. The hormones prevent the ovaries from releasing eggs, keep the lining of the uterus from developing, and cause thickening of cervical mucus, thereby blocking sperm. EFFECTIVENESS: 99%
DEPO-PROVERA®	An injection of synthetic progesterone is given intramuscularly every three months. This inhibits ovulation, thickens cervical mucus, and interferes with implantation. EFFECTIVENESS: >99% if no human error

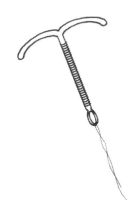

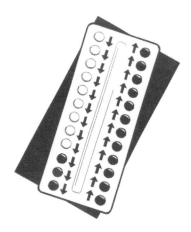

156. SURGICAL METHODS OF CONTRACEPTION

METHOD   **DESCRIPTION**

VASECTOMY   Surgery is performed to cut and tie the vas deferens. There is no sperm in the semen.
                        EFFECTIVENESS: 99–100%

TUBAL LIGATION   The fallopian tubes are blocked by ligation, or by application of rings, bands, or clips, or are cut and tied. The egg and sperm cannot unite.
                        EFFECTIVENESS: 99–100%

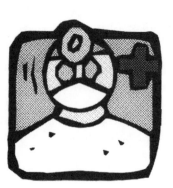

157. ADVANTAGES AND DISADVANTAGES OF CONTRACEPTIVE METHODS

METHOD	ADVANTAGES	DISADVANTAGES
ABSTINENCE	100% protection against pregnancy and STI; no side effects; no cost; may fit religious and personal beliefs	unrealistic for some
IMPLANTS (NORPLANT®)	lasts 5 years; no loss of spontaneity	irregular cycles; high initial cost; no STI protection
DEPO-PROVERA®	lasts 3 months; no loss of spontaneity	irregular cycles; some side effects; no STI protection
ORAL CONTRACEPTIVES	no loss of spontaneity; less bleeding and cramping during periods	irregular cycles; some side effects; must take daily; no STI protection
MALE CONDOM	easy to purchase; protects against STIs	loss of spontaneity; less sensation
FEMALE CONDOM	easy to purchase; protects against STIs	loss of spontaneity; less sensation; messy
SPERMICIDES	easy to purchase; protects against STIs	loss of spontaneity; messy
VASECTOMY	permanent; no loss of spontaneity	permanent; no STI protection
TUBAL LIGATION	permanent; no loss of spontaneity	permanent; no STI protection
IUD	no loss of spontaneity	risk of infection and infertility; increased menstrual bleeding; no STI protection
CERVICAL CAP	used only when needed; protects against STI (when used with spermicide)	must be inserted before intercourse; slight risk of infection
DIAPHRAGM	used only when needed; protects against STI (when used with spermicide)	must be inserted before intercourse; slight risk of infection
FERTILITY AWARENESS	no side effects; low cost; may fit religious and personal beliefs	periods of abstinence; time consuming

Source: Choosing Health High School, *Sexuality & Relationships*. Santa Cruz, CA: ETR Associates, 1997.

158. EFFECTIVENESS OF SOME CONTRACEPTIVE METHODS

Below is a list of the percent of women experiencing a pregnancy within the first year of use:

Method	Perfect Use	Typical Use
Abstinence	0	?
Implants (Norplant®)	.09	.09
Depo-Provera®	.30	.30
Oral Contraceptives	.10	3
Male Condom	3	12
Male Condom with Spermicide	less than 1	5
Female Condom	5	21
Spermicides	6	21
Vasectomy	.10	.15
Tubal Ligation	.40	.40
IUD	1.5	2
Cervical Cap	9	18
Diaphragm	6	18
Fertility Awareness	4	20
No Method	85	85

Source: Hatcher, Robert A., et al. *Contraceptive Technology*, 16th ed. New York: Irvington Publishers, 1994.

159. CURRENT USE AND NONUSE OF CONTRACEPTIVES

More than 3.6 million unplanned pregnancies occur each year. More than half (53%) of all unintended pregnancies are due to nonuse of contraception.

Percentage of Contraceptive Usage by Women Who Intend on Future Births:

➠ No Method   14.6%

➠ Barriers/Spermicides   29.2%

➠ Oral Contraceptives   48.8%

➠ Sterilization   0.2%

➠ Other   7.2%

Percentage of Contraceptive Usage by Women Who Do Not Intend on Future Births:

➠ No Method   6.4%

➠ Barriers/Spermicides   14.9%

➠ Oral Contraceptives   12.1%

➠ Sterilization   61.2%

➠ Other   5.3%

Sources: The Alan Guttmacher Institute for Reproductive Health. The National Center for Health Statistics.

160. LUBRICANTS THAT WEAKEN OR DISINTEGRATE LATEX CONDOMS

If used as a lubricant for sexual intercourse, the following products can weaken or destroy a latex condom. These products *should not* be used with a latex condom.

➠ Cooking Oil

➠ Vegetable Oil

➠ Petroleum Jelly (Vaseline)

➠ Baby Oil

➠ Hand Lotion

➠ Body Lotion

➠ Crisco

➠ Chocolate Syrup

➠ Suntan Lotions or Creams

161. NONMETHODS OF BIRTH CONTROL

The following should not be relied upon as methods of birth control:

WITHDRAWAL

Removal of the penis from the vagina just before ejaculation so that sperm is deposited outside the vagina. This method is not very effective since pre-ejaculatory fluid can contain enough sperm to cause pregnancy.

DOUCHING

Some women douche with water or other special solutions immediately after intercourse in an attempt to remove semen from the vagina before sperm enter the uterus. This does not work because sperm enter the uterus immediately and douching will push some sperm up into the uterus even as it is washing others away.

BREASTFEEDING

Although breastfeeding on demand with no supplementary food for the baby may prevent ovulation, it should not be counted on.

STANDING UP DURING INTER-COURSE

This does not prevent pregnancy.

ASTROLOGICAL BIRTH CONTROL

This does not prevent pregnancy.

AVOIDANCE OF ORGASM BY THE FEMALE

Some believe that in order to conceive, a woman must have an orgasm. This is not true.

162. WHO SHOULD NOT USE ORAL CONTRACEPTIVES

Pharmaceutical companies and doctors recommend that women with any of the following conditions should not use oral contraceptives:

➡ A history of blood clotting or inflammation of the veins caused by any disease or condition

➡ Cancer of the breast or any other reproductive organ

➡ High blood pressure

➡ Liver diseases, such as hepatitis or liver tumors

➡ Undiagnosed abnormal genital bleeding

➡ Very high cholesterol levels

➡ Diabetes mellitus

➡ Smoke 15 cigarettes or more a day and are 35 or older

➡ Pregnancy

➡ Previous cholestasis (obstruction of gall bladder and flow of bile) during pregnancy

Women with these conditions should use oral contraceptives only under a doctor's care:

➡ Very overweight

➡ High risk for heart disease

➡ Migraine headaches or other severe headaches

➡ Slightly increased blood pressure

➡ Impaired liver function

➡ Slightly high cholesterol levels

➡ Have had diabetes in the past

➡ Malignant melanoma (skin cancer)

➡ Meningioma (a cancer of the nervous system)

➡ Congenital hyperbilirubinemia (Gilbert's disease)

➡ A seizure disorder requiring anticonvulsant medication

➡ Smoke several cigarettes per day

➡ Elective major surgery planned within a few weeks

➡ Major surgery that requires immobilization

➡ Long leg casts or injury to the lower leg

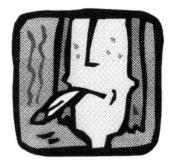

163. RISK OF DEATH ASSOCIATED WITH BIRTH CONTROL METHODS, PREGNANCY, AND ABORTION

	Chance of Death in a Year
Birth Control Pills (nonsmoker)	1 in 63,000
Birth Control Pills (smoker)	1 in 16,000
IUDs	1 in 100,000
Barrier Methods	none
Natural Methods	none
Sterilization:	
Laparoscopic Tubal Ligation	1 in 67,000
Hysterectomy	1 in 1,600
Vasectomy	1 in 300,000
Pregnancy:	
Terminating Pregnancy:	
Illegal Abortion	1 in 3,000
Legal Abortion:	
Before 9 Weeks	1 in 500,000
Between 9–12 Weeks	1 in 67,000
Between 13–16 Weeks	1 in 23,000
After 16 Weeks	1 in 8,700
Continuing Pregnancy	1 in 14,300

Adapted from: Hatcher, Robert A., et al., *Contraceptive Technology,* 1990-1992, 15th rev. ed. New York: Irvington, 1990.

PREGNANCY AND CHILDBIRTH

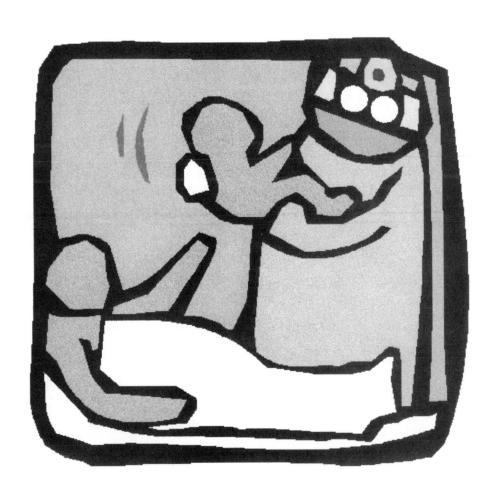

164. GLOSSARY OF PREGNANCY TERMS

ABORTION Spontaneous: A pregnancy loss during the first twenty weeks of pregnancy.

AFTERBIRTH The placenta which is expelled in the final stage of labor.

AID Artificial Insemination Donor.

ANOVULATION Failure to ovulate.

ASSISTED REPRODUCTIVE TECHNOLOGY (ART) Several procedures used to bring about conception without sexual intercourse.

CERVIX The opening between the uterus and the vagina.

CONCEPTION The moment of fertilization.

CORPUS LUTEUM The yellow glandular body formed in the ovary; secretes estrogen and progesterone. These hormones cause the lining of the uterus to thicken in preparation for the reception of the ovum (egg cell).

DONOR INSEMINATION Artificial insemination with donor sperm.

ECTOPIC PREGNANCY A pregnancy outside the uterus, usually in the Fallopian tube.

EGG RETRIEVAL A procedure used to obtain eggs from ovarian follicles for use in in vitro fertilization.

EMBRYO TRANSFER Placing an egg fertilized outside of the uterus into a woman's uterus or Fallopian tube.

ENDOMETRIOSIS A condition in which endometrial tissue is abnormally present outside the uterus or in the abdominal cavity.

EPISIOTOMY An incision made in the perineum to allow passage of the baby's head through the vagina without tearing the vaginal tissue.

ESTROGEN Female sex hormone.

FERTILE Capable of producing offspring.

FERTILIZATION The union of the male sperm and the female ovum (egg).

FRATERNAL TWINS Twins that develop from two separate sperm fertilizing two separate ova (eggs).

GAMETE A reproductive cell: sperm in men, the egg in women.

HUMAN CHORIONIC GONADOTROPIN (HCG) The hormone produced in early pregnancy.

HYSTEROSCOPY	A procedure in which the physician checks for uterine abnormalities by inserting a fiber-optic device.
IDENTICAL TWINS	Twins that develop from a single sperm fertilizing a single ovum (egg) that divides into two zygotes.
IMPLANTATION	The embedding of the embryo in the wall of the uterus.
INFERTILITY	The inability to conceive after a year of unprotected sexual intercourse, or the inability to carry a pregnancy to term.
LACTATION	The production of milk in the mother's breasts following childbirth.
MISCARRIAGE	Spontaneous loss of an embryo or fetus from the womb.
MOTILITY	The ability of sperm to propel themselves to reach the ovum (egg).
OVULATION	The release of the mature egg (ovum) from the ovarian follicle.
PERINEUM	The area of a female between the vaginal opening and the anal opening.
PLACENTA	The embryonic tissue that attaches to the uterine wall and provides a means for exchanging the baby's waste products for the mother's nutrients and oxygen. The baby is connected to the placenta by the umbilical cord.
POSTPARTUM PERIOD	The first few weeks after giving birth.
PROGESTERONE	The hormone produced by the corpus luteum during the second half of a woman's cycle. This hormone thickens the uterine lining to prepare it to accept implantation of a fertilized egg.
PROLACTIN	The hormone that stimulates the production of milk in breast-feeding women.
PREMATURE BIRTH	The birth of a baby before the thirty-seventh week of pregnancy.
STERILITY	An irreversible condition that prevents conception.
STILLBIRTH	The death of a fetus between the twentieth week of pregnancy and birth.
TESTOSTERONE	The male sex hormone.
TRANSITION	The end of the first stage of childbirth.
TUBAL PREGNANCY	The implantation of a fertilized egg in a Fallopian tube.
UMBILICAL CORD	Two arteries and one vein encased in a gelatinous tube leading from the baby to the placenta. This structure is used to exchange nutrients and oxygen from the mother for waste products from the baby.
ZYGOTE	A fertilized egg that has not yet divided.

165. DETECTING PREGNANCY

SIGNS OF PREGNANCY

➡ Missed menstrual period

➡ Tenderness in the breasts

➡ Nausea

➡ Vomiting

➡ Fatigue

➡ Change in appetite

PREGNANCY TESTS

BLOOD TEST

This tests for the presence of HCG (Human Chorionic Gonadotropin) in the blood. In pregnancy, the placenta produces large quantities of HCG, which can be detected in the female's blood as early as 6–8 days after fertilization. The test is performed by a physician.

URINE TEST

HCG is also found in urine and can be detected in as few as 7 days after conception. The test is performed by a physician and is 99 percent accurate.

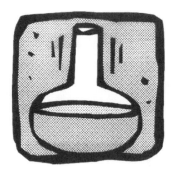

166. FETAL DEVELOPMENT STAGES

Within 36 hours after fertilization, the embryo reaches a two-cell stage. Within two weeks, it becomes implanted in the uterine wall. At that time, heart tissues and blood cells are already developing.

END OF THE 1ST MONTH

➡ Heart begins to beat at 3.5 weeks

➡ Three parts of the brain are formed

➡ Lungs and thyroid gland are developing

➡ Some eye rudiments are present

➡ Measures about 1/4 inch long

END OF THE 2ND MONTH

➡ Brain waves are evident

➡ Spine and nervous system are forming

➡ Heart and circulation are functioning

➡ Limbs are forming, including the beginning of features such as hands and fingers, knees and toes

➡ Measures about 1 to 1-1/2 inches long

END OF THE 3RD MONTH

➡ Muscular development sufficient to open and close mouth and swallow

➡ Skin is evident

➡ Lymph glands develop

➡ Bone marrow makes blood cells

➡ Sex is detectable from the genitals

➡ Placenta is fully formed

➡ Weighs about 1 ounce

➡ Measures about 3 inches long

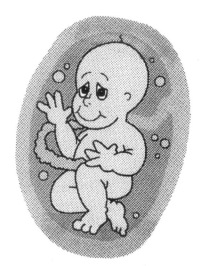

END OF THE 4TH MONTH

➡ Fetus can suck thumb and urinate

➡ Movement can be felt

➡ Face has human features

➡ Weighs about 6 ounces

➡ Measures about 8–10 inches long

END OF THE 5TH MONTH

➡ Fingernails begin to grow

➡ Eyelashes appear

➡ Heartbeat can be heard

➡ Weighs about 1 pound

➡ Measures about 12 inches long

END OF THE 6TH MONTH

➡ Fingernails and toenails are complete

➡ Can cry and kick

➡ Hears sounds

➡ Fetal position changes from 21 to 28 weeks

END OF THE 7TH MONTH

➡ Eyelid can open

➡ Hand can grip

➡ Arms and legs can move

➡ Weighs about 2 to 2-1/2 pounds

END OF THE 8TH MONTH

➡ Hair is growing

➡ Layer of fat develops under skin

➡ Measures about 16 inches long

➡ Weighs about 4 pounds

END OF THE 9TH MONTH

➡ Birth

➡ Organs can function on their own

➡ Measures about 18–20 inches long

➡ Weighs typically 7–9 pounds

167. STAGES OF PREGNANCY

FIRST TRIMESTER   First three months after conception.
                       After month two, the embryo is called a fetus.

SECOND TRIMESTER   Months four to six after conception.

THIRD TRIMESTER   Months seven to nine after conception.

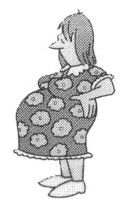

168. A METHOD OF CALCULATING THE DELIVERY DATE

The average length of a human pregnancy is 266 days, or about nine months. A physician is most qualified to calculate the due date. Here is another method:

1. Count back 3 months from the first day of the last menstrual period.

2. Add 7 days plus 1 year to that date.

Example:

If the last menstrual period began on September 10, 1998, the delivery date would be:

September 10, 1998, minus 3 months = June 10, 1998.

June 10, 1998, plus 7 days and 1 year = June 17, 1999.

Source: Education for Sexuality and HIV/AIDS. Blacklick, OH: Meeks Heit Publishing Company, 1993.

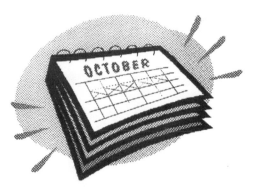

169. DANGER SIGNS DURING PREGNANCY

A pregnant woman should contact her health care provider if any of the following signs or symptoms occur during pregnancy:

➡ Bleeding or leaking of fluid from the vagina

➡ Cramps that are strong

➡ A lasting backache or bellyache

➡ Excessive vomiting or diarrhea

➡ A fever above 100 degrees

➡ Puffy face, fingers, and feet

➡ Prolonged headache

➡ Blurred vision or spots in front of the eyes

➡ Pain or burning during urination

➡ The baby is moving less than usual

Source: March of Dimes Birth Defects Foundation, 1996, White Plains, NY.

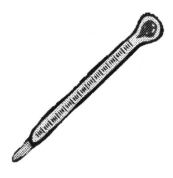

170. THINGS TO AVOID DURING PREGNANCY

DRUGS

➠ Caffeine
➠ Alcohol
➠ Tobacco
➠ Over-the-Counter Drugs (aspirin, cold medications, etc.)
➠ Prescription Drugs
➠ Illicit Drugs

TOXIC SUBSTANCES

➠ Cat Litter Boxes
➠ Solvents (some cleaners or paint thinners)
➠ Lead
➠ Mercury
➠ Insecticides

PROCEDURES

➠ X-Rays

OTHER

➠ Handling uncooked meat
➠ Eating undercooked meat
➠ Saunas, hot tubs, or steam rooms

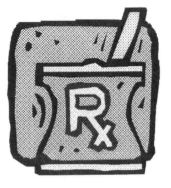

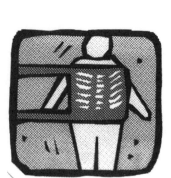

171. SPECIAL FOOD NEEDS DURING PREGNANCY

VITAMINS Take 400 micrograms of the B vitamin folic acid every day before and during pregnancy to reduce the risk of certain birth defects of the brain and spinal cord.
Sources: orange juice, green leafy vegetables, broccoli, fortified breakfast cereals.

IRON See a health care provider about prenatal vitamins containing iron (for healthy blood).

CALCIUM See a health care provider about prenatal vitamins containing calcium (for healthy bones).

BALANCED DIET 6–11 servings of grain products
3–5 servings of vegetables
2–4 servings of fruit
4–6 servings of milk and milk products
3–4 servings of meat and protein foods
Limit fatty foods and sweets

FLUIDS Drink at least 6–8 glasses of water, fruit juice, or milk each day.

Source: March of Dimes Birth Defects Foundation, 1996, White Plains, NY.

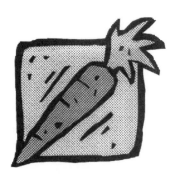
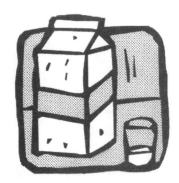
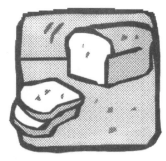
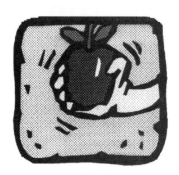
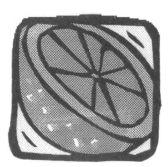

172. ATYPICAL CONDITIONS DURING PREGNANCY

MULTIPLE BIRTHS

Twins	Two babies.
Identical	One egg fertilized by one sperm that divides after fertilization.
Fraternal	Two separate eggs fertilized by two separate sperm.
Triplets	Three babies.
Quadruplets	Four babies.
Quintuplets	Five babies.
Sextuplets	Six babies.
Septuplets	Seven babies.
Conjoined Twins	Twins who are physically joined at birth.

MISCARRIAGE   Also called a spontaneous abortion. Natural expulsion of the embryo or fetus before it has a chance to survive outside the mother.

PREMATURE BIRTH   A baby born before the 37th week of development.

PSEUDOCYESIS   A false pregnancy. Signs and symptoms of pregnancy may be present, but female is not pregnant.

ECTOPIC PREGNANCY   A fertilized ovum implants itself somewhere other than the lining of the uterus.

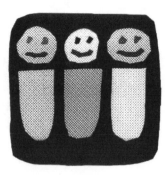

173. CHILDBIRTH PREPARATION METHODS

No longer is childbirth education limited to helping women get through labor without drug assistance; it also allows women to experience labor and delivery with greater knowledge of what is happening to their bodies. Here are some of the methods of childbirth currently taught in childbirth classes:

LAMAZE — The most popular method, Lamaze, combines the psychological with the physical in its approach to handling pain. The theory taught is that knowledge and relaxation techniques combat pain. There are three different breathing patterns for the three stages of labor.

BRADLEY — The Bradley method was the originator of father-coached births and emphasizes diet and exercise. It teaches women to mimic the deep and slow breathing of sleep.

GRANTLY DICK-READ — Grantly Dick-Read focuses on helping a woman overcome fear and tension to build her confidence in her own ability to give birth. This is accomplished through discussions about the process of labor and birth, and how the body works, as well as about diet and exercise. Instruction includes exercises and positions to make the woman more comfortable during labor.

LEBOYER TECHNIQUE — The LeBoyer approach focuses on the birth experience of the infant. It is believed that the baby's transition from the inner world to the outer world should not be traumatic. This method encourages dim lights in the delivery room, soft music, low voices, skin-to-skin contact on the mother's abdomen, and placing the baby in a tub of water at body temperature.

Sources: March Little, Benilde, *YOUR Pregnancy: Giving Birth With Confidence*. Heart & Soul, 1995. *Education for Sexuality and HIV/AIDS*. Blacklick, OH: Meeks Heit Publishing Company, 1993.

174. STAGES OF LABOR AND CHILDBIRTH

DILATION OF THE CERVIX

⟹ Can last from 2 hours to an entire day

⟹ Effacement (thinning out of the cervix) takes place

⟹ Dilation (widening of the cervix) takes place

⟹ Beginning contractions are weak, short, and far apart

⟹ Later contractions become more intense, last longer, and occur more frequently

Transition (End of stage 1)

Cervix enlarges to 8–10 centimeters

Very strong contractions lasting a minute or more

Contractions occur every 1–3 minutes

DELIVERY OF THE BABY

⟹ Baby drops farther down into the birth canal, usually head first

⟹ The mother experiences an urge to push the baby out

⟹ Crowning (head emerging) occurs

⟹ Episiotomy (cut in the perineum) may be performed

⟹ Continued contractions of the uterus deliver the baby

⟹ This stage can last from a few minutes to an hour or more

⟹ Once baby is out and breathing on its own, the umbilical cord is cut

DELIVERY OF THE PLACENTA

⟹ The placenta (afterbirth) is expelled

⟹ The uterus contracts tightly to close off the blood vessels that supplied the placenta through the walls of the uterus

Sources: Education for Sexuality and HIV/AIDS. Blacklick, OH: Meeks Heit Publishing Company, 1993.

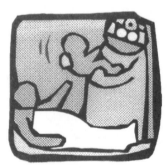

175. PAIN RELIEF DURING CHILDBIRTH

Medications for managing pain are sometimes used during labor and delivery. These drugs can have an adverse effect on the mother, as well as the fetus, and should be avoided whenever possible.

TYPES OF ANESTHESIA

LOCAL
Used to eliminate pain in small, specific areas for short periods of time.

Paracervical Block—no longer recommended.

Pudendal Block—injection of an anesthetic around the nerves on each side of the vagina to numb the perineum and vulva.

REGIONAL
Affects a larger area of the body.

Spinal—injection into the spinal fluid surrounding the lower spinal cord, which numbs the body from the waist down

Epidural—injection into the back (but not into the spinal fluid) that eliminates pain from the waist down, but allows the mother some muscle control

GENERAL
Affects the whole body, creating temporary, but complete, unconsciousness.

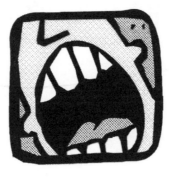

176. APGAR TEST

The APGAR Test, named after the late Dr. Virginia Apgar, is a routine test given one minute after birth and repeated five minutes after birth. The test is used to determine an infant's physical condition at birth. The test measures a baby's condition in five significant areas.

Areas Measured:	Possible Score:
Appearance or Coloring	0–2
Pulse	0–2
Grimace or Reflex Irritability	0–2
Activity	0–2
Respiration	0–2
	0–10

Score Results:

A score of 7–10 is considered normal.

A lower score can be a sign that the baby needs special medical attention.

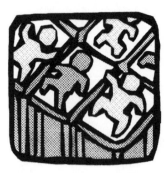

177. ASSISTED REPRODUCTIVE TECHNOLOGY (ART) METHODS

ARTIFICIAL OR INTRAUTERINE INSEMINATION (IUI)

Introduction of semen into the vagina by artificial means so that conception can occur.

IN VITRO FERTILIZATION (IVF)

Mature ova (eggs) are removed from a female's ovary and placed in a lab dish to be fertilized by sperm. After 48–72 hours, the developing embryos are placed directly into the female's uterus so implantation can occur.

GAMETE INTRA-FALLOPIAN TRANSFER (GIFT)

Sperm and ova (eggs) are placed directly in the Fallopian tube, where fertilization takes place naturally.

ZYGOTE INTRA-FALLOPIAN TRANSFER (ZIFT)

Combination of IVF and GIFT. The ova (eggs) and sperm are collected, fertilized in vitro, then placed in the Fallopian tube.

OVA DONATION

Eggs may be donated for artificial insemination and are usually given to females who do not ovulate, do not have ovaries, or do not want to pass on an inherited disease.

EMBRYO FREEZING

During IVF, if more eggs are removed than necessary, the remainder may be frozen for possible future use.

SURROGATE MOTHER

An infertile couple pays a fertile female to be artificially inseminated by the husband's sperm. After the baby is born, the baby is given to the couple for adoption.

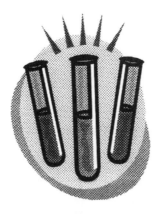

178. LEADING CATEGORIES OF BIRTH DEFECTS

Birth defects are grouped into three major categories: (1) structural/metabolic; (2) congenital infections; and (3) other conditions. The *estimated* incidence of these birth defects is provided below:

Birth Defects	Estimated Incidence
Structural/Metabolic	
Heart & Circulation	1 in 115 births
Muscles & Skeleton	1 in 130 births
Club Foot	1 in 735 births
Cleft lip/palate	1 in 930 births
Genital & Urinary Tract	1 in 135 births
Nervous System & Eye	1 in 235 births
Anencephaly	1 in 8,000 births
Spina Bifida	1 in 2,000 births
Chromosomal Syndromes	1 in 600 births
Down Syndrome (Trisomy 21)	1 in 900 births
Respiratory Tract	1 in 900 births
Metabolic Disorders	1 in 3,500 births
PKU	1 in 12,000 births
Congenital Infections	
Congenital Syphilis	1 in 2,000 births
Congenital HIV Infection	1 in 2,700 births
Congenital Rubella Syndrome	1 in 100,000 births
Other	
Rh Disease	1 in 1,400 births
Fetal Alcohol Syndrome	1 in 1,000 births

Source: March of Dimes Birth Defects Foundation, 1996, White Plains, NY.

179. TESTS TO DETECT BIRTH DEFECTS DURING PREGNANCY

ALPHA-FETOPROTEIN SCREENING

AFP is a substance produced by the liver of the fetus. Some of this protein is excreted into the amniotic fluid and some can be found in the mother's bloodstream. High levels of AFP are associated with neural tube birth defects, such as spina bifida and anencephaly.

AMNIOCENTESIS

Removal of a small amount of amniotic fluid to examine the chromosomes, study the body chemistry, and determine the sex of the fetus. This is usually performed 16 to 20 weeks after conception.

CHORIONIC VILLUS SAMPLING (CVS)

A small piece of membrane from the chorion (a layer of tissue that develops into the placenta) is removed and examined for possible genetic defects. This test takes place around the eighth week of fetal development.

ULTRASOUND

An exam that involves the use of high-density sound waves to form images on a television screen. These images are viewed by a physician.

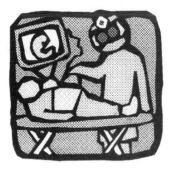

180. BIRTH DEFECTS

Birth defects are the leading cause of infant death and a major cause of disability in young people, affecting more than 150,000 babies each year. Here are some birth defects, their causes, and their descriptions:

PRENATAL

ACCUTANE
This is a prescription medication for severe cystic acne. There is an extremely high risk of fetal malformations if taken during pregnancy.

ALCOHOL
Drinking during pregnancy can cause fetal alcohol syndrome (FAS), a combination of physical and mental birth defects.

CHICKENPOX
This is a mild viral infection characterized by an itchy rash and fever. If the mother contracts chickenpox, the fetus could develop a rare condition called congenital varicella syndrome. This is a group of birth defects that includes blindness, seizures, and mental retardation. Another risk includes a severe chickenpox infection in the newborn.

CHLAMYDIA
This is a sexually transmitted infection that endangers a healthy pregnancy and is linked with miscarriage, low birth weight, and infant death.

COCAINE
Use of this illicit drug during pregnancy can lead to low birth weight, miscarriage, or brain damage in the fetus, and can cause the placenta to pull away from the walls of the uterus, which can cause extensive bleeding. This can be fatal to both the mother and the baby.

CONGENITAL AIDS
Infants infected with HIV suffer frequent infections and diarrhea, fail to thrive or gain weight. Enlarged lymph glands, spleen, liver, and salivary glands are common.

DIABETES
Most women with diabetes can look forward to having a healthy baby. Women with poorly controlled preexisting diabetes are several times more likely than nondiabetic women to have a baby with a serious birth defect, a miscarriage, or a stillbirth.

FIFTH DISEASE
This is a common, usually mild childhood disease that is characterized by a distinctive "slapped cheek" rash. This illness, caused by a virus called parovirus B-19, got its name when it appeared fifth in a list of what were then considered the common causes of rash and fever in childhood. Most fetuses are unaffected when the mother contracts parovirus B-19, but if the fetus does contract it, it can disrupt the fetus' ability to produce red blood cells and possibly lead to miscarriage or stillbirth.

GENITAL HERPES
Mothers who contracted this viral infection can pass it on to their babies. Some infected newborns develop skin or mouth sores or eye infections. Herpes infections in newborns often spread to the brain and many internal organs. About half of these infants die or develop serious brain damage.

| **RUBELLA** | Rubella, also called German measles, is a childhood illness that poses a serious threat to the fetus if the mother contracts the illness during pregnancy. |
| **TOXOPLASMOSIS** | This is a parasitic infection that is widespread in cats and also found in some raw meats. If a woman becomes infected during pregnancy, she risks miscarriage, stillbirth, or infant death soon after birth. |

GENETIC

ACHONDROPLASIA	A genetic disorder of bone growth that is evident at birth.
CLEFT LIP & PALATE	An opening in the lip, roof of the mouth, or the soft tissue in the back of the mouth.
CLUBFOOT	Several kinds of ankle and foot deformities present at birth.
CONGENITAL HEART DEFECTS	Conditions that can affect any of the different parts or functions of the heart.
DOWN SYNDROME	A combination of birth defects including some degree of mental retardation and characteristic facial features. This is caused by an extra # 21 chromosome.
MARFAN SYNDROME	A variable pattern of abnormalities primarily affecting the heart, blood vessels, lungs, eyes, bones, and ligaments.
NEUROFIBROMATOSES	Genetic disorders of the nervous system.
PKU	PKU (Phenylketonuria) is an inherited disorder of body chemistry that, if untreated, causes mental retardation.
RH DISEASE	Rh hemolytic disease of the newborn is a condition caused by incompatibility between the blood of the mother and that of her fetus.
SICKLE CELL DISEASE	An inherited disease that can cause bouts of pain, damage to vital organs, and for some, death in childhood or early adulthood. Most cases in the U.S. occur among African-Americans and Hispanics of Caribbean ancestry.
SPINA BIFIDA	This is often called open spine and is a birth defect of the backbone and sometimes the spinal cord.
TAY-SACHS	Babies with Tay-Sachs disease are born without a blood chemical that is necessary for breaking down certain fatty deposits in brain and nerve cells. Descendants of Central and Eastern European Jews are primarily affected, although members of any group may inherit the disease.
THALASSEMIA	Consists of a group of inherited diseases of the blood.

Source: March of Dimes Birth Defects Foundation, 1996, White Plains, NY.

181. ON AN AVERAGE DAY IN THE UNITED STATES

10,860	Babies are born
1,424	Babies are born to teen mothers
790	Babies are born low birth weight
467	Babies are born to mothers who receive late or no prenatal care
412	Babies are born with a birth defect
145	Babies are born very low birth weight
90	Babies die before reaching their first birthday
20	Babies die as a result of a birth defect

Source: National Center for Health Statistics, 1993 and 1994 final data. Prepared by March of Dimes, 1996.

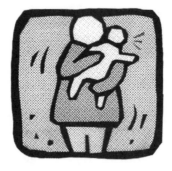

182. IMPACT OF TEEN PREGNANCY

IMPACT ON THE CHILD

➡ A baby born to a first-time teenage mother is more likely to be premature (*Kids Having Kids,* report by the Robin Hood Foundation, 1996)

➡ Low birth weight babies are more common among teenagers. Because of their weight, these babies are 40 times more likely than normal-weight babies to die within their first month of life (March of Dimes Birth Defects Foundation)

➡ A child of an adolescent mother is more likely to be neglected, physically abused, or abandoned (*Kids Having Kids*)

➡ A child of a teenage mother consistently scores lower than children of older mothers on measures of cognitive development (*Sex and America's Teenagers,* The Alan Guttmacher Institute, New York)

➡ A child born to an unmarried, teenage, high school dropout is 10 times more likely to live in poverty than a child born to a mother who is married, out of her teens, and graduated from high school (*Kids Count, 1996,* The Annie E. Casey Foundation)

➡ A child of a single teen mother is more likely to drop out of school, give birth outside of marriage, divorce or separate, and become dependent on welfare (*Kids Count, 1996*)

➡ The daughter of an adolescent mother is up to 83 percent more likely to become a teenage mother herself (*Kids Having Kids*)

➡ The son of an adolescent mother is 2.7 times more likely to be arrested and imprisoned than the son of a mother who delayed childbearing until her early twenties (*Kids Having Kids*)

IMPACT ON THE MOTHER

➡ More than 80 percent of teen mothers become impoverished and dependent on welfare (*Kids Having Kids*)

➡ Only about three in every 10 adolescent mothers earn a high school diploma by the age of 30 (*Kids Having Kids*)

➡ During the first 13 years of parenthood, adolescents earn an average of about $5,600 annually, which is less than half the poverty level (*Kids Having Kids*)

IMPACT ON OUR SOCIETY

➡ Adolescent childbearing costs U.S. taxpayers an estimated $6.9 billion each year due to increased medical care expenses, welfare, and food stamps (*Kids Having Kids*)

➡ When all subsequent consequences of adolescent pregnancy are considered, the gross annual cost is an estimated $34 billion (*Kids Having Kids*)

➡ An estimated 53 percent of funds dispersed by Aid to Families With Dependent Children (AFDC), the most common form of welfare, goes to families formed by a teenage birth (ADFC)

➡ Adolescent childbearing costs taxpayers roughly $1 billion each year to build and maintain prisons for the sons of young mothers (*Kids Having Kids*)

Source: Teen Pregnancy Fact Sheet (Campaign for Our Children).

183. TEEN PREGNANCY STATISTICS

TEENAGE PREGNANCY

➡ More than 1 million U.S. teenagers become pregnant each year

➡ 1 in 5 women who are aged 15-19 and who are sexually active become pregnant each year

➡ Nonwhite teenagers have twice the pregnancy rate of white teenagers

➡ Approximately 50 percent of teenage pregnancies result in birth, 36 percent in an abortion, and an estimated 14 percent in miscarriage

➡ By age 18, one in four young women (24%) will have a pregnancy

➡ Nearly one in five teenagers who experience a premarital pregnancy will get pregnant again within a year

➡ Eight in ten teenage pregnancies are unintended

➡ U.S. teenagers have one of the highest pregnancy rates in the western world

TEENAGE CHILDBEARING

➡ About half of all teenage pregnancies end in birth

➡ More than nine in 10 teenagers who give birth keep their babies; few place their babies for adoption

➡ On average, 33 percent of women under age 20 who give birth receive inadequate prenatal care, either because they start care late in their pregnancy or they have too few medical visits

TEENAGE ABORTION

➡ Four in 10 teenage pregnancies (excluding miscarriages) end in abortion

➡ 26 percent of all abortions in the U.S. each year are to women under age 20

➡ Every year, about 4 percent of women aged 15–19 have an abortion

➡ The top three reasons cited by pregnant teenagers for choosing to have an abortion were concern about how having a baby would change their lives, their feeling that they are not mature enough to have a child, and financial problems

➡ Many states currently have mandatory parental consent or notice, or professional counseling laws in effect for a minor to obtain an abortion

Source: Pregnancy and Childbearing Among U.S. Teens. Planned Parenthood Federation of America, Inc., 1993.

184. PREGNANCY OPTIONS

1. HAVE THE BABY AND RAISE THE CHILD

➠ Raise the child with a partner

➠ Raise the child without a partner

2. HAVE THE BABY AND PLACE THE BABY FOR ADOPTION

CLOSED ADOPTION   The names of the birth mother and the adoptive parents are kept secret from each other.

OPEN ADOPTION   The birth mother may select the adoptive parents for her child.

Adoption is arranged in three ways:

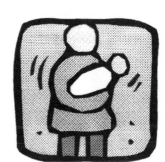

Agency Adoption—Child is placed through a public or private agency that is licensed by the government.

Independent Adoption—adoption is arranged through a doctor or lawyer, or someone else who knows a couple who wishes to adopt.

Adoption by Relatives—adoption within the mother's own family. Must still be approved by a family- or surrogate-court judge.

FOSTER CARE   In some cities and counties, temporary foster care may be available for the children of mothers who need more time to decide between adoption and parenting.

3. END THE PREGNANCY

ABORTION   A medical procedure that removes the embryo or fetus from the uterus, usually by vacuum suction.

185. TYPES OF ABORTIONS

MEDICAL ABORTIONS

Use of a combination of drugs to terminate a pregnancy.

Two Types of Drugs:

➡ *Methotrexate-Misoprostol Method*—a woman receives an injection of methotrexate from her clinician. Five to seven days later she returns and inserts suppositories of misoprostol into her vagina. The pregnancy usually ends at home within a day or two.

➡ *Mifepristone-Misoprostol Method*—a woman swallows a dose of mifepristone under the guidance of her clinician. She returns in several days and inserts suppositories of misoprostol into her vagina. The pregnancy usually ends at home within four hours.

EARLY ABORTIONS

(6–14 weeks after the last menstrual period)

➡ *Suction Curettage*—the cervix is dilated and a tube is inserted into the uterus. This tube is attached to a suction machine. The uterus is emptied by gentle suction. After the suction tube has been removed, a curette (narrow metal loop) may be used to scrape the walls of the uterus to be sure that it is completely emptied.

EARLY SECOND TRIMESTER

(Available up to the 24th week of pregnancy)

➡ *Dilation and Evacuation (D & E)*—the fetus and tissue are removed from the uterus with instruments and suction curettage.

ABORTION AFTER 24 WEEKS

➡ *Induction Method*—the doctor injects urea or salt solution into the uterus to induce contractions (labor) and cause a stillbirth. Or the doctor may insert prostaglandin into the vagina to induce labor and expel the fetus.

➡ *Three Step D & E Procedure*—the cervix is dilated several times until it is wide enough to allow the removal of the fetus with grasping instruments.

RELATIONSHIPS AND COMMUNICATION

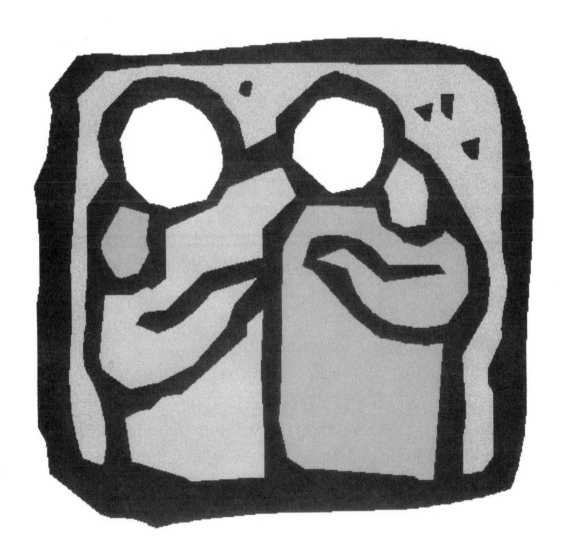

186. TYPES OF COMMUNICATION

Communication refers to the many ways people send and receive information.

VERBAL COMMUNICATION   The use of language and words to convey a message. Includes speaking skills and listening skills.

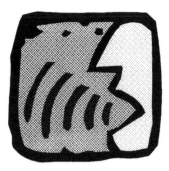

NONVERBAL   Communication without using words. Includes the use of symbols, signs, or body language to convey a message.

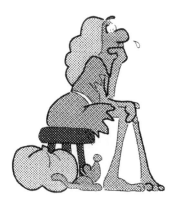

187. LEVELS OF COMMUNICATION

*People can communicate with each other on many different levels
depending on their relationship and the situation.
Five levels of communication are described below:*

1. CLICHÉ CONVERSATION

➠ Lowest level of communication in which a person rarely shares any feelings or information about himself or herself. Includes small talk such as, "How are you?" and "Fine, and you?"

2. GIVING INFORMATION AND REPORTING FACTS

➠ Involves reporting events without opinions and feelings.

3. EXPRESSING IDEAS

➠ At this level, people begin to share information about themselves, so there is more risk involved.

4. SHARING FEELINGS

➠ Moves toward a state of emotional understanding. Instead of just expressing ideas about a situation, people begin to express how the situation makes them feel.

5. SELF-DISCLOSURE

➠ Is the highest level of communication, reserved for intimate relationships between friends, family, and partners. Characterized by sharing of each other's happiness, sadness, fears, joys, and other emotions.

Adapted from: Kranzler, Nora J., and Kathleen R. Miner, *Health Facts: Self-Esteem & Mental Health.* Santa Cruz, CA: ETR Associates, 1994.

188. BARRIERS TO GOOD COMMUNICATION

These conditions may interfere with good communication:

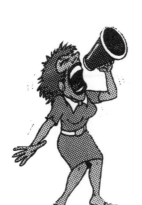

➡ Unclear explanations
➡ Conflicting messages
➡ Not listening
➡ Personal biases
➡ Interrupting
➡ Blaming or yelling
➡ Assuming you understand
➡ Bringing up the past
➡ Using guilt trips
➡ Using profane language
➡ Giving unwanted advice
➡ Mocking or ridiculing another person
➡ Using violence

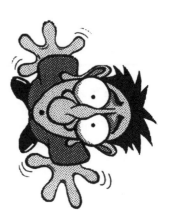

189. COMMUNICATION STOPPERS

These conditions usually stop or slow down communication:

INTERRUPTING — Butting in as the person tries to talk.

CHALLENGING/ CONTRADICTING — Questioning everything the speaker has to say.

DOMINATING — Taking over the conversation.

JUDGING — Evaluating everything the speaker has to say.

ADVISING — Giving a lot of unwanted advice.

INTERPRETING — Analyzing everything in order to find its "deeper meaning."

PROBING — Asking question after question in a demanding tone.

CRITICIZING/ PUT-DOWNS — Making sarcastic, negative remarks about the speaker or the speaker's feelings and ideas.

190. REFUSAL SKILLS

Suggestions on how to say "No":

1. DECIDE AHEAD OF TIME

If possible, decide ahead of time how you feel about something (drugs, sex, etc.), and stick to it. You have control over your choices. Don't allow someone else to make decisions for you.

2. BE FRIENDLY, YET FIRM

It is possible to be assertive and confident without being snobbish.

3. BE HONEST

You should not have to lie to avoid doing something you don't want to do or don't think is right. Simply state the truth and leave it at that.

4. SPEAK ONLY FOR YOURSELF

You are not responsible for everyone else's actions. Don't feel that you must tell others what to do (unless they are harming you or someone else). Simply refuse to participate.

5. SUGGEST AN ALTERNATIVE

If you feel uncomfortable or don't wish to do something, suggest an alternative. (Ex: "I don't want a beer; I'd like a Coke instead.")

6. AFFIRM THE PERSON

Separate the activity from the person. Let the person know that you still care about her or him, but you don't want to participate in the activity.

7. APPEAL TO POSSIBLE CONSEQUENCES

If someone asks you to break the law or do something that makes you uncomfortable, explain the possible consequences and your feelings about those consequences.

8. ACCEPT THE POSSIBILITY OF REJECTION

Even if you decline graciously and don't condemn your friends, someone may resent and reject you anyway. You must determine if this is truly a friendship.

191. STYLES OF REFUSING

Refusal skills are those techniques and strategies that you can learn to help you say no effectively when you are faced with something that is against your morals or that you do not want to do. The styles of refusing that people use are listed below:

PASSIVE METHOD   Give up or give in, without standing up for your own rights or beliefs.

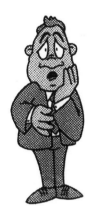

AGGRESSIVE METHOD   Be overly forceful, pushy, hostile, and demanding.

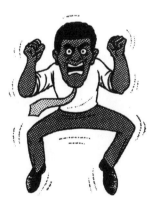

ASSERTIVE METHOD   Stand up for your own rights in a firm but positive manner. You state your position, acknowledge the rights of the other individual, then stand your ground.

192. RELATIONSHIP SKILLS

RELATIONSHIP SKILLS FOR STUDENTS TO DEVELOP:

➠ Practicing active listening
➠ Initiating a conversation
➠ Maintaining a conversation
➠ Ending a conversation
➠ Joining others in an activity
➠ Introducing people
➠ Understanding feelings of others
➠ Expressing friendship
➠ Helping others
➠ Coping with feeling left out
➠ Dealing with contradictory messages
➠ Responding to teasing
➠ Requesting desired action when appropriate
➠ Using "I Messages" when appropriate
➠ Building loyalty and trust by keeping confidences
➠ Setting limits when appropriate

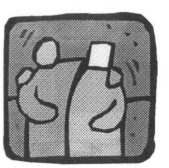

RELATIONSHIP SKILLS WITH ADULTS:

➠ Requesting help
➠ Requesting permission
➠ Demonstrating responsibility
➠ Negotiating privileges
➠ Requesting reconsideration

193. THE THREE COMPONENTS OF A RELATIONSHIP

INTIMACY   Feelings of closeness and "connectedness" that are experienced in loving relationships.

PASSION   The drive that leads to romance, physical attraction and sexual interaction. Passion involves a high degree of physical arousal and an intense desire to be with the other person.

COMMITMENT   A decision that one person cares for another and wants to maintain the relationship.

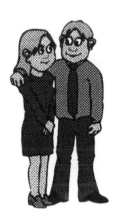

194. CONSTRUCTIVE ELEMENTS IN A RELATIONSHIP

⇒ Honesty

⇒ Trust

⇒ Open communication

⇒ Personal self-esteem

⇒ Responsibility for self

⇒ Dependability

⇒ Flexibility

⇒ Patience

⇒ Thoughtfulness

195. DESTRUCTIVE ELEMENTS IN A RELATIONSHIP

➡ Abuse

➡ Desire to control

➡ Dishonesty or deceitfulness

➡ Jealousy

➡ Impatience

➡ Lack of self-esteem

➡ Overdependency

➡ Selfishness

196. SIGNS OF TROUBLED RELATIONSHIPS

➡ Changes in communication

➡ Continued unresolved conflicts

➡ Insufficient amount of quality time spent together

➡ Emotional, physical or verbal abuse

➡ Ignorance of the other's needs

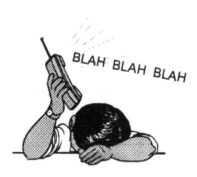

197. REASONS FOR ENDING RELATIONSHIPS

➡ Abuse
➡ Alcohol or other drug addiction or abuse
➡ Unmet expectations
➡ Differences in sexual desires or rules
➡ Lack of physical attraction
➡ Lack of common interests
➡ Change in feelings about the other person
➡ Moving away
➡ Loss of job, income, financial stability
➡ Infidelity
➡ Loss of trust
➡ Possessiveness of partner
➡ Family pressures
➡ Friendship pressures
➡ Religious differences
➡ Age differences
➡ Unmet needs

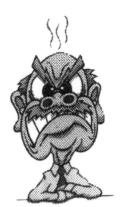

198. TYPES OF FAMILIES

NUCLEAR FAMILY   Parents and one or more children sharing a household.

SINGLE-PARENT FAMILY   Only one parent living with the child or children.

EXTENDED FAMILY   One or more relatives in addition to the nuclear family or single-parent family.

BLENDED FAMILY   A type of nuclear family in which one or both people have been married before.

ADOPTIVE FAMILY   Through a legal procedure, one or more of the children have become a part of the family through adoption.

FOSTER FAMILY   Through special arrangements with governmental agencies or foster parent and child organizations, the children are cared for by a particular family.

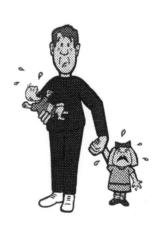

199. THE FIVE MOST COMMON MAJOR FAMILY CRISES

➼ Financial Problems
➼ Divorce
➼ Drug Use
➼ Violence
➼ Death

200. FACTORS AFFECTING MARITAL RELATIONSHIPS

According to various studies, the following factors are indicators of a well-adjusted marriage— one in which both members have adapted well to married life and to each other.

➼ Having the same or similar values
➼ Agreeing on important issues
➼ Showing affection
➼ Sharing common interests
➼ Sharing confidences
➼ Complaining rarely about the marriage
➼ Not feeling lonely or irritable

201. SOCIAL BACKGROUND FACTORS OF SUCCESSFUL MARITAL RELATIONSHIPS

➼ Sharing similar family backgrounds
➼ Seeing parental happiness at home
➼ Not experiencing conflict with parents
➼ Having a close friendship before marriage
➼ Associating with friends of both sexes
➼ Both partners experiencing educational achievement
➼ Having occupational security and stability
➼ Participating in outside organizations and associations

202. COMMUNICATION AND RELATIONSHIP FACTS

➡ About 25 million families with children include a mother and a father, while 8 million have a mother only, and 2 million have a father only, according to 1997 Census Bureau figures

➡ Of the 30 million households without families, 83% consist of one person living alone

➡ In 1987, statistics showed that approximately one million adolescents ran away from home every year. Estimates are now as high as two million. Most are victims of abuse.

➡ The incidence of divorce has steadily increased in America since World War II with the divorce rate doubling between 1970 and 1980

➡ Approximately half of all children have experienced family disruption through divorce

➡ About 2/3 of all adolescent admissions to psychiatric hospitals are children who have experienced divorce in the family

➡ In 1996, about 55% of men and 52% of women aged 15 and older were married, according to U.S. government statistics for 1996

➡ Of all women who divorce before the age of 25, 81% are likely to remarry

➡ Every year, about 100,000 people call off their weddings

➡ Approximately 10% of adults remain single for life

➡ About 11% of families were below the official government poverty level in 1995

➡ The average television viewing time of teens, ages 12 to 17, is about 10 hours a week, according to a Nielsen Media Research report for May 1997; the heaviest viewing time is from 4:30 to 7:30 pm, Monday through Friday, when the group logs in three hours.

➡ One friendship survey shows that most people have between one and five good friends

➡ More than 3,000 languages are spoken in the world today

➡ Students spend about 60% of a typical school day in listening and about 15% in speaking

STRESS MANAGEMENT AND SELF-ESTEEM

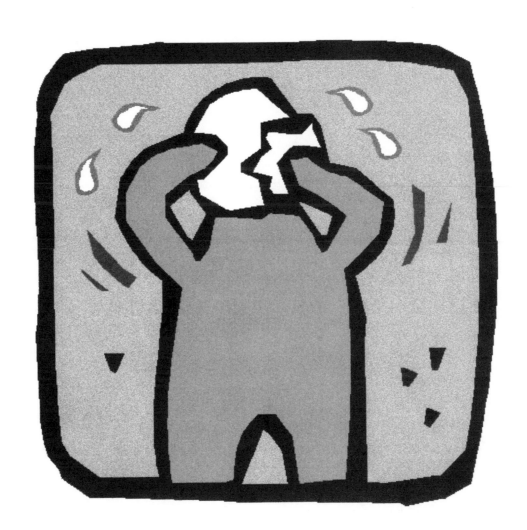

203. MAJOR CAUSES OF STRESS FOR ADULTS AND TEENS

Stress occurs when the pressures upon us exceed our abilities to cope with those pressures.

ADULTS

➤ Illness
➤ Job changes
➤ Moving
➤ Separation
➤ Deaths in the family
➤ Financial difficulties
➤ Marriage
➤ Arrival of a baby

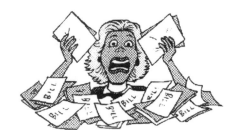

TEENS

➤ Feelings about themselves
➤ Feelings about peers
➤ Conflict with parents
➤ Pressures at school

204. ADOLESCENT LIFE-CHANGE-EVENT STRESSORS

Each life-change event, listed below from most to least stressful, can threaten one's sense of security. These stressors may result from both positive and negative change.

1. Being pregnant and unwed
2. Death of a parent
3. Death of a sister or brother
4. Death of a friend
5. Divorce or separation of parents
6. Becoming an unwed father
7. Becoming involved with alcohol or other drugs
8. Family member's alcohol or other drug problem
9. Having a parent go to jail for a year or more
10. Having a change in acceptance by peers
11. Discovering that you are adopted
12. Loss or death of a pet
13. Having a parent remarry
14. Having a visible deformity
15. Having a serious illness that requires hospitalization
16. Going to a new school
17. Moving to a new home
18. Failing a grade in school
19. Not making a team or extracurricular activity
20. Having a parent become seriously ill
21. Beginning to date
22. Being suspended from school
23. Having a newborn brother or sister
24. Arguing more with parents
25. Having an outstanding personal achievement
26. Parents arguing more
27. Having a parent lose his or her job
28. A change in parents' financial status
29. Being accepted to college
30. Having a brother or sister leave home
31. Death of a grandparent
32. Having a grandparent move in
33. Marriage of a brother or sister

205. FACTORS INFLUENCING STRESS

The variation in the impact of a stressor on a person is related to the person's age, social status, income, state of health, diet, sleep habits, cultural background, and previous experience.

EXTERNAL DEMANDS

➠ Family
➠ Individual
➠ Social
➠ Environmental
➠ Financial
➠ Work/school

INTERNAL DEMANDS

➠ Responsibility
➠ Obligations
➠ Self-criticism

VULNERABILITY

➠ Genetic predisposition
➠ Coping skills
➠ Lifestyle

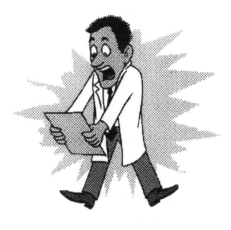

SYMPTOMS/ILLNESS

ATTITUDES/BELIEFS/VALUES

PAST EXPERIENCES

A person's response to a stressor also varies depending on how much control that person thinks that he or she has over a situation.

CHRONIC STRESSES—stressors that continue indefinitely or are recurrent.

MAJOR LIFE EVENTS—stressors that are bad for a period of time and then go away.

DAILY HASSLES—unpleasant, often temporary, events.

206. EFFECTS OF STRESS ON HEALTH AND THE BODY

COMMON PHYSICAL SYMPTOMS

⇒ Muscle tension

⇒ Headaches

⇒ Low back pain

⇒ Insomnia

⇒ High blood pressure

MAJOR CONTRIBUTING FACTOR TO:

⇒ Coronary artery disease

⇒ Cancer

⇒ Respiratory disorders

⇒ Accidental injuries

⇒ Cirrhosis of the liver

⇒ Suicide

AGGRAVATES:

⇒ Multiple sclerosis

⇒ Diabetes

⇒ Herpes

⇒ Mental illness

⇒ Alcoholism

⇒ Drug abuse

⇒ Family discord and violence

Source: National Mental Health Association, 1998, Washington, DC.

207. GUIDELINES FOR COPING WITH STRESS

The National Mental Health Association recommends the following strategies for coping with stress:

➡ If you feel overwhelmed by some activities (yours and/or your family's) learn to say "NO"

➡ Eliminate an activity that is not absolutely necessary, or ask someone else to help

➡ Be willing to listen to others' suggestions, and be ready to compromise

➡ Don't expect perfection from yourself or others

➡ Take time to listen to music, relax, and try to think of pleasant things or nothing at all

➡ Use your imagination, and picture how you can manage a stressful situation more successfully

➡ Take one thing at a time

➡ Exercise. Twenty to thirty minutes of physical activity benefits both the body and the mind.

➡ Take a break from your worries by doing something you enjoy

➡ Limit intake of caffeine and alcohol (alcohol actually disturbs, not helps, regular sleep patterns), get adequate rest, exercise, and balance work and play

➡ Let friends and family provide love, support, and guidance—don't try to cope alone

➡ Make allowances for others' opinions and be prepared to compromise

➡ Go easy with criticism. You may expect too much of yourself and others.

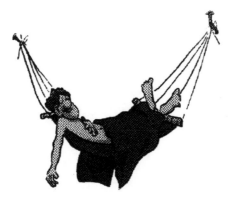

208. HELPFUL HINTS FOR REDUCING STRESS DURING TEST TAKING

LEARN THE MATERIAL TO BE COVERED BY THE TEST

➠ Examine the syllabus

➠ Talk to the instructor

➠ Look at old tests

➠ Consult with other students

➠ Use textbook/workbook

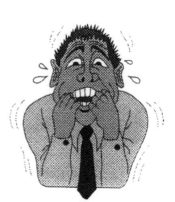

GATHER AND ORGANIZE THE SUPPLIES NEEDED FOR THE TEST

➠ Have working pens or sharpened pencils

➠ Check to make sure your calculator is working

➠ Take a watch to the exam

PAY ATTENTION TO NUTRITIONAL AND SLEEP REQUIREMENTS BEFORE A TEST

➠ Get a good night's sleep each day for several days before the test

➠ Exercise or do something fun to burn off extra energy

➠ Eat a balanced meal before the test

➠ A high carbohydrate dinner the night before helps to raise energy levels

➠ Get a drink of water before the test

➠ Avoid excessive amounts of caffeine

➠ Dress in layers so that you may adjust to changes in temperature

CONCENTRATE ON ATTITUDE AND MOTIVATION

➠ Focus on past testing success

➠ Engage in positive self talk

Source: Muskingum College, Center for Advancement of Learning, Learning Strategies Database.

209. SIGNS OF HIGH AND LOW SELF-ESTEEM

High Self-Esteem

➠ Having an internal locus of control, gaining approval from within, rather than outside of self

➠ Ability to balance extremes in one's thinking, feeling, and acting. Learning from mistakes and being able to say, "I made a mistake; I'm sorry."

➠ Taking responsibility for own perceptions and reactions and not projecting onto others

➠ Ability to listen to inner self and act on this guidance

➠ Having self-respect, self-confidence, and self-acceptance

➠ Having awareness of one's strengths and weaknesses

➠ Knowing areas of self to be improved and what needs to be accepted

➠ Growing and taking positive risks

Low Self-Esteem

➠ Extremes in thoughts, feelings, and behaviors

➠ Self-blame and self-criticism or constant blame and fault finding of others

➠ Over- or under-achieving or eating

➠ Staying a victim—not taking responsibility for positive changes

➠ Fear of change and risk taking

➠ Negative thinking—or so optimistic that reality is denied

➠ Constant emotional reaction to others

➠ Bragging and pushing self on others

➠ Demanding to be right, needing to have agreement or have one's own way most of the time

Source: National Mental Health Association, 1998, Washington, DC.

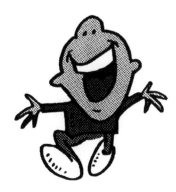

210. SKILLS FOR IMPROVING SELF-ESTEEM

➡ Understand your own personal significance in school, family, and community

➡ Recognize your personal capabilities in all areas—intellectual, physical, social, emotional and more

➡ Make lists of your skills, talents and qualities and review them often

➡ Examine your specific, creative talents and use them regularly

➡ Set realistic and attainable goals for yourself, base your goals on improvement, not perfection

➡ Don't consider your weaknesses without considering your strengths

➡ Believe in your ability to influence your own life

➡ Seek training or instruction in a special area of interest

➡ Stay in school and seek help for areas in which you experience problems

➡ Practice skills that help you relate to others such as identifying and expressing your feelings and being sympathetic toward others' feelings

➡ Practice the inner skills of exercising self-control and self-discipline

➡ Make friends with others who respect you and are likely to approve of you and accept you as an individual

➡ Build a network of friends

➡ Care about yourself; practice good health and safety

➡ Reject negative signs or comments from others intended to make you feel bad

➡ Connect your own personal decisions and actions to consequences and results

➡ Accept errors or mistakes as steps in learning and attaining goals instead of looking at them as signs of failure

➡ Visualize successful situations

➡ Celebrate your successes, even the small ones; give yourself credit

211. GUIDELINES FOR GOAL SETTING

SPECIFIC: Set a goal that has a definite result.

REALISTIC: Set a goal you can reach.

CHALLENGING: Make your goal interesting.

CONCRETE: Make your goal something that can be measured.

SELF-REFERENCED: Focus your goals based upon what you can do.

Source: *Wrestle to Win!,* Hendrix, Beasey, Ed. S., High Performance Athletics, P.O. Box 669364, Marietta, GA 30066, 1996.

212. TIME-MANAGEMENT TECHNIQUES FOR STUDENTS

STUDY WHEN:

- Plan two study hours for every hour you spend in class
- Study difficult (or boring) subjects first
- Avoid scheduling marathon study sessions
- Be aware of your best time of day
- Use waiting time
- Use a regular study area

STUDY WHERE:

- Choose a place that minimizes visual and auditory distractions
- Use the library
- Don't get too comfortable. Sit (or even stand) so that you can remain awake and attentive.
- Find a better place when productivity falls off

YOU AND THE OUTSIDE WORLD:

- Pay attention to your attention
- Agree with family about study time
- Avoid noise distractions
- Get off the phone
- Learn to say "No"
- Hang a "Do Not Disturb!" sign on your door
- Ask: "What is one task I can accomplish toward my goal?"
- Ask: "Am I beating myself up?" (Lighten up, don't berate self).
- Ask: "Am I too much of a perfectionist?"
- Ask: "How did I just waste time?"
- Ask: "Would I pay myself for what I'm doing right now?"
- Ask: "Can I do just one more thing?" (Stretch yourself)

Source: Gregory Wells, Coordinator, William James Center, Davis and Elkins College. Elkins, WV, NACADA Conf. 1987.

213. ABRAHAM MASLOW'S HIERARCHY OF NEEDS

American psychologist, Abraham Maslow, developed a ranked order of needs that human beings must have in order to survive and grow. The most basic physical needs such as hunger and thirst must be satisfied before a human being becomes aware of and is able to meet additional emotional needs such as love and recognition.

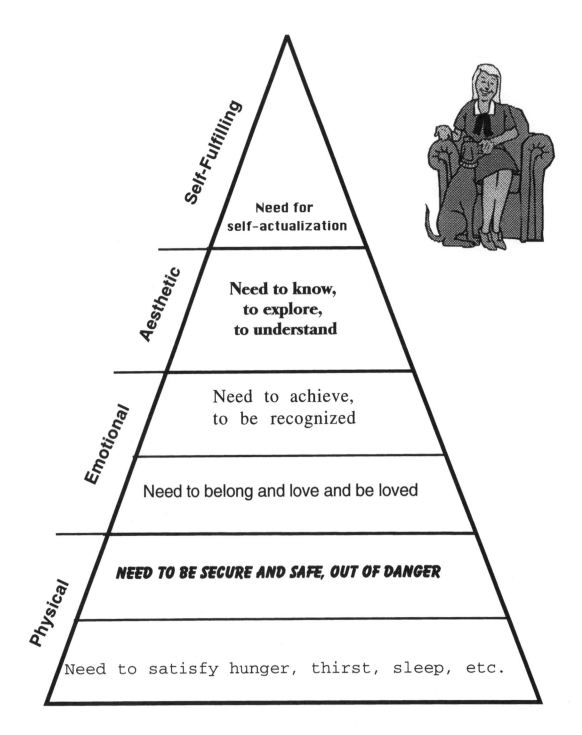

Self-Fulfilling

Aesthetic

Emotional

Physical

Need for
self-actualization

**Need to know,
to explore,
to understand**

Need to achieve,
to be recognized

Need to belong and love and be loved

NEED TO BE SECURE AND SAFE, OUT OF DANGER

Need to satisfy hunger, thirst, sleep, etc.

214. CATEGORIES OF PHOBIAS

Psychiatry identifies three different types of phobias:

AGORAPHOBIA

➡ Irrational anxiety about being in places from which escape might be difficult or embarrassing

SOCIAL PHOBIA

➡ Irrational anxiety elicited by exposure to certain types of social or performance situations, also leading to avoidance behavior

SPECIFIC PHOBIA

➡ Persistent and irrational fear in the presence of some specific stimulus, which commonly elicits avoidance of that stimulus, that is, withdrawal

215. COMMON PHOBIAS

➡ Acrophobia—Fear of heights

➡ Aerophobia—Fear of flying

➡ Agoraphobia—Fear of open spaces or of being in crowded places

➡ Algophobia—Fear of pain

➡ Arachnephobia—Fear of spiders

➡ Autophobia—Fear of being alone

➡ Bibliophobia—Fear of books

➡ Brontophobia—Fear of thunder

➡ Claustrophobia—Fear of closed spaces

➡ Lygophobia—Fear of darkness

➡ Murophobia—Fear of mice

➡ Panaphobia—Fear of everything

➡ Paraskavedekatriaphobia—Fear of Friday the 13th

➡ Pyrophobia—Fear of fire

➡ Zoophobia—Fear of animals

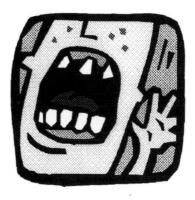

216.   HEALTHFUL WAYS TO DEAL WITH ANGER

Expressing anger in safe, nondestructive ways can help to reduce the risk of hurting yourself or someone else.

➡ Channel your energies into productive work or recreational activities

➡ Get away by yourself

➡ Have a good cry

➡ Do hard physical exercise

➡ Punch a pillow or punching bag

➡ Count to ten slowly. Take a deep breath as you do, and then slowly exhale to the count of ten.

➡ Call a friend and talk it out

➡ Close your eyes and listen to good music

➡ Write down exactly how you are feeling and why—no one needs to see what you write

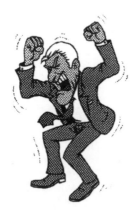 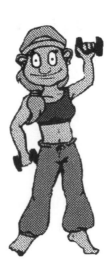

217. TYPES OF MENTAL AND PERSONALITY DISORDERS

PERSONALITY DISORDERS

ANTISOCIAL PERSONALITY DISORDER

Characterized by a long-standing pattern of a disregard for other people's rights.

AVOIDANT PERSONALITY DISORDER

Characterized by a long-standing and complex pattern of feelings of inadequacy, extreme sensitivity to what other people think about them, and social inhibition.

BORDERLINE PERSONALITY DISORDER

Characterized by unstable interpersonal relationships.

DEPENDENT PERSONALITY DISORDER

Characterized by a long-standing need for the person to be taken care of and a fear of being abandoned or separated from important individuals in his or her life.

HISTRIONIC PERSONALITY DISORDER

Characterized by a pattern of excessive emotionality and attention seeking.

NARCISSISTIC PERSONALITY DISORDER

Characterized by a need for admiration, and lack of empathy.

OBSESSIVE-COMPULSIVE PERSONALITY DISORDER

Characterized by a pattern of preoccupation with orderliness, perfectionism, and mental and interpersonal control, at the expense of flexibility, openness, and efficiency.

SCHIZOID PERSONALITY DISORDER

Characterized by a pattern of detachment from social relationships and a restricted range of expression of emotions in interpersonal relationships.

PARANOID PERSONALITY DISORDER

Characterized by a pervasive distrust and suspicion of others.

SCHIZOTYPAL PERSONALITY DISORDER

Characterized by a pattern of social and interpersonal deficits marked by eccentric behaviors and a discomfort with close relationships.

MENTAL DISORDERS

ANOREXIA NERVOSA A life-threatening eating disorder defined by a refusal to maintain body weight within 13 percent of an individual's minimal normal weight.

ANXIETY DISORDERS

PANIC DISORDER Characterized by panic attacks, panic disorder results in sudden feelings of terror that strike repeatedly and without warning.

OBSESSIVE-COMPULSIVE DISORDER (OCD) OCD is characterized by repeated, intrusive, and unwanted thoughts (obsessions) and/or rituals that seem impossible to control (compulsions).

POST-TRAUMATIC STRESS DISORDER Persistent symptoms of this disorder occur after experiencing a trauma such as abuse, natural disasters, or extreme violence.

PHOBIAS A phobia is a disabling and irrational fear of something that really poses little or no actual danger.

GENERALIZED ANXIETY DISORDER Chronic, exaggerated worry about everyday, routine life events and activities that lasts at least six months.

ATTENTION DEFICIT/HYPERACTIVITY DISORDER (ADHD)

➡ Characterized by inattention, impulsivity, and hyperactivity. Although children and adolescents with ADHD may not perform well in school, the disorder does not signal a lack of intelligence.

MANIC-DEPRESSIVE ILLNESS

➡ Also known as bipolar disorder, this is a brain disorder involving episodes of serious mania and depression. The person's mood usually swings from overly "high" and irritable to sad and hopeless, and then back again, with periods of normal mood in between.

DISSOCIATIVE DISORDERS

➡ A dissociation from or interruption of a person's fundamental aspects of waking consciousness, triggered as a response to trauma or abuse.

DEPRESSION

➡ Major depression, or unipolar depression, is manifested by a combination of symptoms that interfere with the ability to work, sleep, eat, and enjoy once-pleasurable activities. It is more than a passing case of the "blues." People with depression cannot just "pull themselves together."

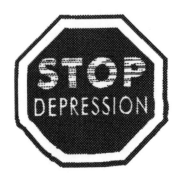

© 1999 by The Center for Applied Research in Education

SEASONAL AFFECTIVE DISORDER (SAD)

➟ A condition marked by seasonal depression, primarily affecting women.

SCHIZOPHRENIA

➟ A serious brain disorder, which affects how a person thinks, feels, and acts. It is a disease that makes it difficult for a person to tell the difference between real and imagined experiences, or to think logically.

SCHIZO-AFFECTIVE DISORDER

➟ Presence of psychotic symptoms in the absence of mood changes for at least two weeks in a patient who has a mood disorder. This is an appropriate diagnosis when the person does not fit diagnostic standards for either schizophrenia or "affective" (mood) disorders such as depression and manic depression.

SLEEP DISORDERS (INSOMNIA)

➟ The inability to get the amount of sleep needed to function efficiently during the day. May be associated with an organic disease (e.g., arthritis, heart disorder), may be a symptom of depression, or may be caused by a person's lifestyle. Sleep disorders are associated with increased mortality, poor career performance, overeating, and increased hospitalization.

TOURETTE'S SYNDROME (TS)

➟ A neurologic syndrome. The essential features of Tourette's are multiple tics that are sudden, rapid, recurrent, nonrhythmic, stereotypical, purposeless movements or vocalizations.

Criteria Summarized from: Diagnostic and Statistical Manual of Mental Disorders, 4th ed. Washington, DC: American Psychiatric Association, 1994.

218. WARNING SIGNS OF MENTAL ILLNESS

The National Mental Health Association lists the following warning signs of mental illness:

YOUNGER CHILDREN

➠ Changes in school performance
➠ Poor grades despite strong efforts
➠ Excessive worry or anxiety (i.e., refusing to go to bed or school)
➠ Hyperactivity
➠ Persistent nightmares
➠ Persistent disobedience or aggression
➠ Frequent temper tantrums

OLDER CHILDREN AND PRE-ADOLESCENTS

➠ Substance abuse
➠ Inability to cope with problems and daily activities
➠ Change in sleeping and/or eating habits
➠ Excessive complaints of physical ailments
➠ Defiance of authority, truancy, theft, and/or vandalism
➠ Intense fear of weight gain
➠ Prolonged negative mood, often accompanied by poor appetite or thoughts of death
➠ Frequent outbursts of anger

ADULT

➠ Confused thinking
➠ Prolonged depression (sadness or irritability)
➠ Feelings of extreme highs and lows
➠ Excessive fears, worries, and anxieties
➠ Social withdrawal
➠ Dramatic changes in eating or sleeping habits
➠ Strong feelings of anger
➠ Delusions or hallucinations
➠ Growing inability to cope with daily problems and activities
➠ Suicidal thoughts
➠ Denial of obvious problems
➠ Numerous unexplained physical ailments
➠ Substance abuse

219. TYPES OF SCHIZOPHRENIA

➡ Paranoid schizophrenia—person feels extremely suspicious, persecuted, or grandiose, or experiences a combination of these emotions

➡ Disorganized schizophrenia—person is often incoherent, but may not have delusions

➡ Catatonic schizophrenia—person is withdrawn, mute, negative, and often assumes very unusual postures

➡ Residual schizophrenia—person is no longer delusional or hallucinating, but has no motivation or interest in life. These symptoms can be most devastating.

220. COMMON SIGNS OF SCHIZOPHRENIA

According to the National Mental Health Association, initial symptoms of schizophrenia may include:

➡ mild feelings of tension

➡ inability to sleep or concentrate

➡ loss of interest in schoolwork and friends

As the disease becomes worse, the individual may experience more disabling and bizarre symptoms such as:

➡ delusions

➡ hallucinations

➡ disordered speech and thoughts

The behavior of children and teens with schizophrenia may differ from that of adults with this illness.

Early Warning Signs:

➡ trouble discerning dreams from reality

➡ seeing things and hearing voices that are not real

➡ confused thinking

➡ vivid and bizarre thoughts and ideas

➡ extreme moodiness

➡ peculiar behavior

➡ concept that people are "out to get them"

➡ behaving younger than chronological age

➡ severe anxiety and fearfulness

➡ confusing television or movies with reality

➡ severe problems in making and keeping friends

221. COMMON SYMPTOMS OF DEPRESSION

➧ A persistent sad, anxious, or "empty" mood

➧ Sleeping too little or sleeping too much

➧ Reduced appetite and weight loss, or increased appetite and weight gain

➧ Loss of interest or pleasure in activities once enjoyed

➧ Restlessness or irritability

➧ Persistent physical symptoms that do not respond to treatment (such as headaches, chronic pain, or constipation and other digestive disorders)

➧ Difficulty concentrating, remembering, or making decisions

➧ Fatigue or loss of energy

➧ Feeling guilty, hopeless, or worthless

➧ Thoughts of death or suicide

These symptoms may indicate depression in adolescence, particularly when they last for more than two weeks:

➧ Poor performance in school

➧ Withdrawal from friends and activities

➧ Sadness and hopelessness

➧ Lack of enthusiasm, energy, or motivation

➧ Anger and rage

➧ Overreaction to criticism

➧ Feelings of being unable to satisfy ideals

➧ Poor self-esteem or guilt

➧ Indecision, lack of concentration, or forgetfulness

➧ Restlessness and agitation

➧ Changes in eating or sleeping patterns

➧ Substance abuse

➧ Problems with authority

➧ Suicidal thoughts or actions

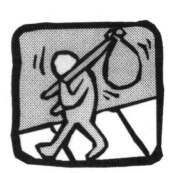

Source: National Mental Health Association, 1998, Washington, DC.

222. HEALTHFUL WAYS TO DEAL WITH EMOTIONS

➡ Recognize an emotion by noticing your body's signals such as

    heart beating faster

    breathing faster or becoming out of breath

    feeling hot or cold

    feeling the stomach or back tighten up

    face getting red or feeling hot

    hands or muscles tightening up

➡ Identify the emotion and what happened to make you feel it

➡ Find a word to label your emotion or feeling

➡ Share the feeling with someone who can be objective

➡ Use an "I message" in describing your feelings

➡ Listen to what the other person has to say

➡ Consider ways to control strong feelings before acting out. These could include some of the following:

    using a pillow or punching bag

    going for a walk

    getting a drink of water

    counting to 25

    visualizing a favorite place or activity

    using some relaxation techniques

    reading or playing a game

➡ Remember that the feeling will eventually go away. If it stays with you for too long, seek help.

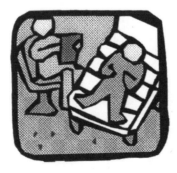

223. TYPES OF MENTAL HEALTH PROFESSIONALS

PSYCHIATRIST — Medical doctor with special training in the diagnosis and treatment of mental and emotional illnesses. Like other doctors, psychiatrists are qualified to prescribe medication.

CHILD/ADOLESCENT PSYCHIATRIST — Medical doctor with special training in the diagnosis and treatment of emotional and behavioral problems in children. Child/Adolescent psychiatrists are qualified to prescribe medication.

PSYCHOLOGIST — Counselor with an advanced degree from an accredited graduate program in psychology, and two or more years of supervised work experience. Trained to make diagnoses and provide individual and group therapy.

CLINICAL SOCIAL WORKER — Counselor with a master's degree in social work from an accredited graduate program. Trained to make diagnoses and provide individual and group counseling.

LICENSED PROFESSIONAL COUNSELOR — Counselor with a master's degree in psychology, counseling, or a related field. Trained to diagnose and provide individual and group counseling.

MENTAL HEALTH COUNSELOR — Counselor with a master's degree and several years of supervised clinical work experience. Trained to diagnose and provide individual and group counseling.

CERTIFIED ALCOHOL AND DRUG ABUSE COUNSELOR — Counselor with specific clinical training in alcohol and drug abuse. Trained to diagnose and provide individual and group counseling.

NURSE PSYCHO-THERAPIST — A registered nurse who is trained in the practice of psychiatric and mental health nursing. Trained to diagnose and provide individual and group counseling.

MARITAL AND FAMILY THERAPIST — A counselor with a master's degree, with special education and training in marital and family therapy. Trained to diagnose and provide individual and group counseling.

PASTORAL THERAPIST — Clergy with training in clinical pastoral education. Trained to diagnose and provide individual and group counseling.

Source: National Mental Health Association, 1998, Washington, DC.

224. TYPES OF TREATMENT FOR MENTAL ILLNESS

According to the National Mental Health Association, psychotherapy is a method of talking face to face with a therapist. The following are a few of the types of available therapy:

BEHAVIOR THERAPY
Includes stress management, biofeedback and relaxation training to change thinking patterns and behavior.

PSYCHOANALYSIS
Long-term therapy meant to "uncover" unconscious motivations and early patterns to resolve issues and to become aware of how those motivations influence present actions and feelings.

COGNITIVE THERAPY
Seeks to identify and correct thinking patterns that can lead to troublesome feelings and behavior.

FAMILY THERAPY
Includes discussion and problem-solving sessions with every member of the family.

MOVEMENT/ART/ MUSIC THERAPY
Includes the use of movement, art, or music to express emotions; effective for persons who cannot otherwise express feelings.

GROUP THERAPY
Includes a small group of people who, with the guidance of a trained therapist, discuss individual issues and help each other with problems.

DRUG THERAPY
Can be beneficial to some persons with mental or emotional disorders.

ELECTRIC CONVULSIVE TREATMENT (ECT)
Used to treat some cases of major depression, delusions, and hallucinations, or life-threatening sleep and eating disorders that cannot be effectively treated with drugs and/or psychotherapy.

225. CHARACTERISTICS OF GOOD MENTAL HEALTH

Psychologically healthy individuals share many of the following characteristics:

⮕ Possess a strong sense of self-acceptance and self-love but are not self-obsessed

⮕ Are aware of their true feelings and motives

⮕ Have confidence in themselves

⮕ Can function independently when they need to and be assertive when they want to be assertive

⮕ Believe that they are basically in control of their lives

⮕ Feel capable of accomplishing their goals

⮕ Possess a clear perception of reality

⮕ Are typically on the optimistic side

⮕ Can find the courage to confront their own fears

⮕ Can accept responsibility (or lack of it) for their behavior

⮕ Are prepared to take risks when it is reasonable to do so

⮕ Are able to adapt to new situations and "bounce back" after crises and setbacks

⮕ Live "balanced" lives and are rarely extremists, fanatics, or gluttons

⮕ Have the capacity and desire to care deeply about the welfare of another person, persons, and/or humanity in general

⮕ Truly appreciate and enjoy various aspects of life

⮕ Are generally active, curious, and enthusiastic

⮕ Have found meaning and purpose in their lives

⮕ Are committed to something outside of themselves

226. SOURCES OF MENTAL-HEALTH SUPPORT AND INFORMATION

➡ Family physician

➡ Clergyperson

➡ Family services agencies, such as Catholic Charities, Family Services, or Jewish Social Services

➡ Educational consultants or school counselors

➡ Marriage and family counselors

➡ Child guidance counselors

➡ Psychiatric hospitals accredited by the Joint Commission on Accreditation of Health Care Organizations

➡ Hotlines, crisis centers, and emergency rooms (call Directory Assistance)

➡ Your local health department's Mental Health Division

➡ Other mental health organizations

FOR INFORMATION CONTACT:

NATIONAL MENTAL HEALTH ASSOCIATION
1021 Prince Street
Alexandria, VA 22314
Phone: 800-969-6642
http://www.nmha.org

CENTER FOR MENTAL HEALTH SERVICES (CMHS)
Knowledge Exchange Network
5600 Fishers Lane, Room 13-103
Rockville, MD 20857
Phone 800-789-2647

AMERICAN PSYCHOLOGICAL ASSOCIATION
750 First Street, NE
Washington, DC 20002
Phone 800-374-2721 or 202-336-5500

NATIONAL ALLIANCE FOR THE MENTALLY ILL (NAMI)
200 N. Glebe Road, Suite 1015
Arlington, VA 22203-3457
Phone 800-950-6264 (800-950-NAMI)

AMERICAN PSYCHIATRIC ASSOCIATION
1400 K Street, NW
Washington, DC 20005
Phone 202-682-6000

NATIONAL INSTITUTE OF MENTAL HEALTH (NIMH)
Information Resources and Inquiries Branch
5600 Fishers Lane, Room 7C-02
Rockville, MD 20857
Phone 301-443-4513

THE AMERICAN STRESS INSTITUTE
124 Park Avenue
Yonkers, NY 10703
Phone 914-963-1200

NATIONAL ALLIANCE FOR RESEARCH ON SCHIZOPHRENIA
AND DEPRESSION (NARSAD)
60 Cutter Mill Road, Ste 200
Great Neck, NY 11021
Phone 800-829-8289

AMERICAN ACADEMY FOR CHILD AND ADOLESCENT PSYCHIATRY
3615 Wisconsin Avenue NW
Washington, DC 20016
Phone: 800-333-7636

AMERICAN ASSOCIATION OF SUICIDOLOGY
4201 Connecticut Avenue NW, Suite 310
Washington, DC 20008
Phone: 202-237-2280

ANXIETY DISORDERS ASSOCIATION OF AMERICA
6000 Executive Boulevard
Rockville, MD 20852
Phone 301-231-9350

SECTION 12

VIOLENCE PREVENTION

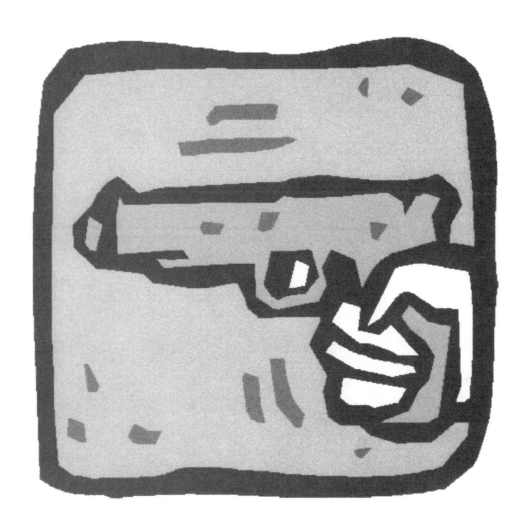

227. REASONS FOR TEEN VIOLENCE

The following are some possible reasons that violence continues in our society:

Loss of "Connectedness"

➡ Many Americans feel isolated from other people due to parents working, kids staying home alone, neighbors not knowing neighbors, etc. Some psychologists feel that this contributes to a self-centered attitude that can turn into violence when someone gets in the way.

Lack of Family Support and Control

➡ According to the Carnegie Council on Adolescent Development, today's teens spend less time with parents and other adults than they did just a few decades ago, and more time watching television or with their peers in unsupervised environments. Unfortunately, some parents are not providing the warmth, guidance, or discipline that helps kids grow into connected, caring adults.

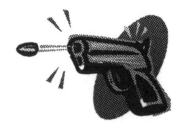

Media Influences

➡ The media portrays violence as glamorous, easy, and attractive, and an everyday occurrence.

Teen Subcultures/Guns

➡ Violent behavior is often a way of gaining respect within teen gangs. Combine that with the easy availability of guns, and you have the ingredients for violence.

Alcohol, Other Drugs, and Risk-Taking

➡ According to some psychologists, mind-altering substances tend to bring our strongest emotions to the surface. For some teens, the strongest emotions are anger and rage. Using alcohol and other drugs is often part of a pattern of violent, risk-taking behavior.

Poverty

➡ Studies show that murder rates soar in neighborhoods where men have no jobs and women struggle to raise children alone.

Adapted from: "When Violence Comes to School," Current Health, Volume 24, No. 8. April/May 1998.

220   Section 12

228. TYPES OF VIOLENCE

ABUSE OR CHILD ABUSE   Harmful treatment of a person under 18—includes physical abuse, sexual abuse, and neglect.

ASSAULT   Physical attack or threat of an attack.

BULLYING   Attempting to hurt or frighten people who are perceived to be smaller or weaker.

DOMESTIC VIOLENCE   Violence occurring within the family or within other relationships of people living together.

FIGHTING   Taking part in a physical struggle.

HOMICIDE   Accidental or purposeful killing of another person.

RAPE   Threatened or actual use of physical force to get someone to have sex without giving consent.

SEXUAL HARASSMENT   Unwanted sexual behavior that ranges from making unwanted sexual comments to forcing another person into unwanted sex acts.

SUICIDE   Intentional taking of one's own life.

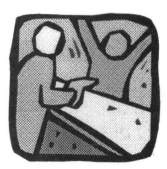

229. FACTS ABOUT GIRLS AND VIOLENCE

According to the Pacific Center for Violence Prevention, juvenile girls are understudied in violence prevention; therefore, accurate data regarding girls and violence are difficult to capture. The following facts about girls are representative of the best statistics available:

IN THE NATION

➡ Homicide is the second leading cause of death of females 15-19 years old.[1]

➡ Homicide is the leading cause of death of African-American females 15-19 years old.[2]

➡ Girls are sexually abused almost three times more often than boys.[3]

➡ Victims of rape are disproportionately children and adolescent girls—60% of forcible rapes occur before the victim is 18 years old; 29% of victims are younger than 11 years old when raped.[4]

➡ Of all rapes and sexual assaults, 75% involve family members, relatives, or acquaintances; 22% involve strangers; and 3% have an uncertain or undetermined relationship.[5]

➡ Of girls involved in the juvenile justice system, 40-70% have a past history of family abuse (physical, sexual, or emotional) compared to 23-34% of girls in the general population.[6]

➡ Girls accounted for 25% of all juvenile arrests in 1994, an increase of 40% from 1985.[7]

➡ Girls accounted for 14% of all juvenile violent crime index arrests in 1994, an increase of 11% from 1985.[8]

➡ Girls are most frequently arrested for nonviolent delinquent offenses such as larceny-theft (usually shoplifting), and for status offenses, in particular, running away from home. In fact, girls are arrested for running away more often than boys, accounting for 57% of such arrests in 1994, even though boys and girls run away from home at similar rates.[9]

➡ Girls were detained and formally charged in juvenile court in 15% of the delinquent offense cases and 42% of the status offense cases in 1992. In particular, girls were detained and formally charged in court more often than boys for running away, accounting for 62% of such cases in 1992.[10]

➡ Although delinquent crime among girls is generally nonviolent in nature, arrest rates for violent crime index offenses committed by girls increased by 125% from 1985 through 1994, while the rates for boys increased 67%. The rate increases among girls were primarily due to rises in arrests for robbery and aggravated assault.[11]

➡ Simple assault (141%), motor vehicle theft (113%), and weapons violation (137%) arrest rates among juvenile girls also increased significantly from 1985 through 1994.[12]

References

[1] Gardner P, Rosenberg HM, Wilson RW. Leading Causes of Death by Age, Sex, Race, and Hispanic Origin: United States, 1992. National Center for Health Statistics. Vital Health Stat 20(29), 1996.

[2] Ibid.

[3] Sedlak AJ, Broadhurst DD. Executive Summary of the Third National Incidence Study of Child Abuse and Neglect. Administration for Children and Families, U.S. Department of Health and Human Services, September, 1996, p. 2. http://www.calib.com/nccanch/data/nis3.txt (15 Nov. 1996).

[4] Rape in America: A Report to the Nation, Arlington, VA.: The National Victim Center, 1992, p. 3.

[5] Ibid, p. 4; Bureau of Justice Statistics, Sex Offenses and Offenders (An Analysis of Data on Rape and Sexual Assault.) NCJ-163392. Washington D.C.: U.S. Department of Justice, 1997. This same Bureau of Justice Statistics report also cites recent FBI data suggesting that 90% of rape victims younger than 12 know the offender. These data, though preliminary, are, nevertheless, compelling.

[6] Prevention and Parity: Girls in Juvenile Justice. Indianapolis, IN: Girls Incorporated, 1996, p. iv.

[7] Snyder HN, Sickmund M, Poe-Yamagata E. Juvenile Offenders and Victims: 1996 Update on Violence. Washington D.C.: Office of Juvenile Justice and Delinquency Prevention, U.S. Department of Justice, 1996, p. 10.

[8] Ibid, p. 11. Federal violent crime index offenses are: criminal homicide, forcible rape, robbery and aggravated assault.

[9] Ibid. Chesney-Lind M, Shelden RG. Girls, Delinquency and Juvenile Justice. Wadsworth Publishing Co.: Belmont, CA. 1992, p. 14. Status offenses (juvenile offenses that would not be crimes if committed by an adult) are: running away from home, curfew violation, truancy, ungovernability (beyond the control of parents or custodians), underage drinking, and smoking tobacco.

[10] Snyder HN, Sickmund M. Juvenile Offenders and Victims: A National Report. Washington, D.C.: Office of Juvenile Justice and Delinquency Prevention, U.S. Department of Justice, 1995, p. 139.

[11] Snyder HN, Sickmund M, Poe-Yamagata E. Juvenile Offenders and Victims: 1996 Update on Violence. Washington D.C.: Office of Juvenile Justice and Delinquency Prevention, U.S. Department of Justice, 1996, p. 11.

[12] Ibid.

Source: Pacific Center for Violence Prevention.

230. THE COST OF VIOLENCE

The direct and indirect costs to Americans of both property and violent crimes are $425 billion each year according to a Business Week report on the cost of all crime in the U.S.

This total of $425 billion exceeds the amount of the $300 billion U.S. national defense budget.

*The $425 billion estimate breaks down as follows:

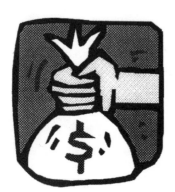

Criminal Justice	*$90 billion* Spending on police, courts, and prisons
Private Protection	*$65 billion* Spending on alarms, private guards, and security systems
Urban Decay	*$50 billion* Cost of lost jobs and fleeing residents
Property Loss	*$45 billion* Value of damaged and stolen goods
Medical Care	*$5 billion* Cost of treating crime victims
Shattered Lives	*$170 billion* Cost of productivity losses and lost quality of life[1]

The lifetime costs for all persons aged twelve and older who are injured due to rape, robbery, assault, arson, and murder in a single year are estimated to be $178 billion.[2]

*The breakdown of the $178 billion estimate is:

Total Monetary	*$23.8 billion* Medical ($2.3 billion) Emergency Services ($219 million) Productivity ($20.6 billion) Administrative ($730 million)
Total Mental Health	*$76.6 billion* Mental Health Medical ($7.2 billion) Mental Health Productivity ($2.7 billion) Quality of Life Lost to Psychological Injury ($66.8 billion)
Quality of Life	*$77.9 billion*[3]

References

[1] Farrell C, The Economics of Crime. Business Week. December 13, 1993. pp. 72-80.

[2] Miller TR, Cohen MA, Rossman SB. Victim Costs of Violent Crime and Resulting Injuries. Health Affairs. 1993;12 (4): 195-197.

[3] Ibid.

Source: Pacific Center for Violence Prevention.

231. COST OF FIREARM-RELATED VIOLENCE

➡ Acute medical care for patients with firearm-related injuries has been estimated to cost nearly $32,000 per hospital admission.[1]

➡ Gunshot wounds are costly. Treatment of gunshot wounds is, on average, twice as expensive as treatment of stab wounds or other intentional injuries.[2]

➡ 80% of the medical cost for treatment of firearm-related injuries is paid for by tax-payers.[3]

➡ Youth gunshot victims in California incurred nearly $50,000,000 in hospital bills, for the initial hospitalization only, in 1992.[4]

➡ Gunshot injuries in California cost $329 million in 1991. Just over half of this cost is for hospitalizations; 44% for other medical care; and 5% for related nonmedical care.[5]

References

[1] Kizer, K.W., Vassar, M.J., Harry, R.L., Layton, K.D. Hospitalization charges, costs, and income for firearm related injuries at a university trauma center. JAMA, 273 (22) June 14, 1995: 1768-1773.

[2] Tellez, M.G, Mackersie, R.C., Morabito, D., Shagoury, C., Heye, C. Risks, costs, and the expected complication of re-injury. Am J Surg, 170 (6) Dec, 1995: 660-664.

[3] Wintemute, G.J., Wright, M.A. Initial and Subsequent Hospital Costs of Firearm Injuries, J Trauma, 33 (4) Oct. 1992: 556-660.

[4] Emergency Preparedness and Injury Control (EPIC) Branch. Violent Injuries to California Youth, Sacramento, CA: California Department of Health Services, September 1996, Report No. 7, Table D-2.

[5] Max, Wendy. The Impact of Gun Violence on California's Health Care System. Testimony before California Assembly Select Committee on Gun Violence, Nov. 29, 1994.

© 1999 by The Center for Applied Research in Education

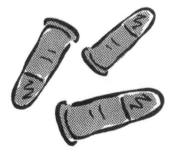

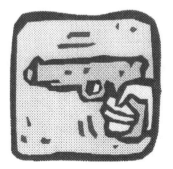

Source: Pacific Center for Violence Prevention. 1996. Permission is granted to distribute this document in unaltered format.

232. FACTS ABOUT YOUTH INCARCERATION

According to the Pacific Center for Violence Prevention, incarceration data are complex and difficult to interpret. Listed below are some of the best available statistics:

GLOSSARY OF TERMS

ADMISSIONS	Number of admissions to a facility regardless of length of stay (for example, the stay could be as short as a single day). This number does not reflect the number of individuals, and could include numerous admissions for a single individual.
ONE DAY COUNTS	The number of individuals in a facility on a given day.
PUBLIC AND PRIVATE FACILITIES	Includes detention centers, shelters, reception/diagnostic centers, training schools, ranch, camp, or farm, halfway houses, or group homes.
INCARCERATION	Includes juveniles detained or committed.
JUVENILE	Refers to youth under 18.

➡ There were 867,527 juvenile admissions to public and private facilities for delinquents in the U.S. in 1994.[1]

➡ 6,408 girls and 53,846 boys were incarcerated in public juvenile facilities in 1993, based on a one day count in public facilities. Girls accounted for 11% of youth in custody. 12% of girls in custody (versus 27% of boys) had committed violent crimes. 12% of girls (versus 1% of boys) were in custody for status offenses (offenses such as truancy, running away and violating curfews that are offenses only because they are committed by juveniles).[2]

➡ Most juvenile commitments to a juvenile correctional agency are for non-violent offenses. 28.1% of juveniles committed in 1994 were violent offenders while 71.9% were non-violent offenders.[3]

➡ Most youth don't return to court. 60% of juveniles referred to juvenile court for the first time never return on a new charge.[4]

References

[1] National Council on Crime and Delinquency. Juveniles Taken into Custody Research Program, Sponsored by the U.S. Department of Justice. Total Admissions for Public and Private Facilities, 1994. Note these are admissions and don't represent 867,527 individuals. See glossary above.

[2] Girls Incorporated National Resource Center & Office of Juvenile Justice and Delinquency Prevention. Prevention and Parity: Girls in Juvenile Justice. Indianapolis, IN: Girls Incorporated, June 1996, p. 6. Incarceration data is based on one day counts in public facilities.

[3] Camp, George M. and Camille Graham. The Corrections Yearbook, 1995. South Salem, NY: Criminal Justice Institute, 1995, p. 22. (Twenty-nine state agencies reported data.)

[4] National Center for Juvenile Justice. NCCJ In Brief, March 1997. Volume 1, No. 3, p. 1.

Source: Pacific Center for Violence Prevention.

233. SEXUAL HARASSMENT DEFINITIONS

COERCE	Use intimidation, threats, or force to make a person behave a certain way.
DISCRIMINATION	Treating a person differently because of the person's race, religion, gender, sexual orientation, or disability; prejudice.
EXPLICIT	Clear, direct, straightforward.
EXPLOIT	Use someone or something for your own personal gain.
GENDER	Being male or female; one's sex.
GENDER ROLE STEREOTYPING	Expecting men and women to behave a certain way because of their gender.
HARASS	Bother, annoy, intimidate, threaten, or scare another person.
IMPLICIT	Not clear; implied, suggested or hinted at.
INTENT	Reason for saying or doing something.
LIABILITY	Legal responsibility or obligation.
PHYSICAL SEXUAL CONDUCT	Touching another person in a sexual way.
SEX OBJECT	Someone who is seen only as an object of sexual desire, not as a person.
SEXISM	Discrimination based on gender.
SEXUAL ADVANCES	Attempts to lure someone into a sexual act.
SEXUAL FAVORS	Sexual acts performed in return for rewards.
SEXUAL HARASSMENT	Unwelcome sexual advances, requests for sexual favors, and other verbal or physical conduct of a sexual nature.
SUBMIT	Go along with something because you have to, not because you wish to.
VERBAL SEXUAL CONDUCT	Sexual comments about a person's body, clothing, gender, and so forth.

234. FACTS ABOUT SEXUAL ASSAULT

The following facts about sexual assault were compiled by the American Medical Association:

INCIDENCE

➡ Sexual assault continues to represent the most rapidly growing violent crime in America.[1]

➡ Over 700,000 women are sexually assaulted each year.[2]

➡ It is estimated that fewer than 50% of rapes are reported.[1]

➡ Approximately 20% of sexual assaults against women are perpetrated by assailants unknown to the victim. The remainder are committed by friends, acquaintances, intimates, and family members. Acquaintance rape is particularly common among adolescent victims.[12]

➡ Male victims represent five percent of reported sexual assaults.[11]

➡ Among female rape victims, 61% are under age 18.[3, 11]

➡ At least 20% of adult women, 15% of college women and 12% of adolescent women have experienced some form of sexual abuse or assault during their lifetimes.[4]

SOCIETAL ATTITUDES

➡ A survey of 6,159 college students enrolled at 32 institutions in the U.S. found:[4]

54% of the women surveyed had been the victims of some form of sexual abuse; more than one in four college-aged women had been the victim of rape or attempted rape;

57% of the assaults occurred on dates;

73% of the assailants and 55% of the victims had used alcohol or other drugs prior to the assault;

25% of the men surveyed admitted some degree of sexually aggressive behavior;

42% of the victims told no one.

➡ In a survey of high school students, 56% of the girls and 76% of the boys believed forced sex was acceptable under some circumstances.[5]

➡ A survey of 11-to-14-year-olds found:[5]

51% of the boys and 41% of the girls said forced sex was acceptable if the boy, "spent a lot of money" on the girl;

31% of the boys and 32% of the girls said it was acceptable for a man to rape a woman with past sexual experience;

87% of boys and 79% of girls said sexual assault was acceptable if the man and the woman were married;

65% of the boys and 47% of the girls said it was acceptable for a boy to rape a girl if they had been dating for more than six months.

➡ In a survey of male college students:

35% anonymously admitted that, under certain circumstances, they would commit rape if they believed they could get away with it.

One in 12 admitted to committing acts that met the legal definitions of rape, and 84% of men who committed rape did not label it as rape.[6, 7]

➡ In another survey of college males:[8]

43% of college-aged men admitted to using coercive behavior to have sex, including ignoring a woman's protest, using physical aggression, and forcing intercourse.

15% acknowledged they had committed acquaintance rape; 11% acknowledged using physical restraints to force a woman to have sex.

➡ Women with a history of rape or attempted rape during adolescence were almost twice as likely to experience a sexual assault during college, and were three times as likely to be victimized by a husband.[9]

➡ Sexual assault is reported by 33% to 46% of women who are being physically assaulted by their husbands.[10]

Sources:

1. Dupre, A.R., Hampton, H.L., Morrison, H., and Meeks, G.R. Sexual Assault. Obstetrical and Gynecological Survey. 1993;48:640-648.

2. National Crime Center and Crime Victims Research and Treatment Center. Rape in America: A Report to the Nation. Arlington, VA; 1992: 1-16

3. National Victim Center, and Crime Victims Research and Treatment Center. Rape in America: A Report to the Nation. Arlington, VA; 1992: 1-16.

4. Koss M.P., Hidden rape: sexual aggression and victimization in a national sample of students in higher education. In: Burgess A.W., ed Rape and Sexual Assault. New York, NY: Garland Publishing: 1988;2:3-25.

5. White, Jacqueline W. and John A. Humphrey. "Young People's Attitudes Toward Acquaintance Rape." Acquaintance Rape: The Hidden crime." John Wiley and Sons, 1991.

6. Koss M.P., Dinero, T.E., Seibel, C.A. Stranger and acquaintance rape: Are there differences in the victim's experience? Psychology of Women Quarterly. 1988: 12: 1-24.

7. Malamuth N.M. Rape proclivity among males. J Soc Issues. 1981;37: 138-157.

8. Rapaport, Karen R. and C. Dale Posey. Sexually Coercive College Males. Acquaintance Rap The Hidden Crime, edited by Andrea Parrot. John Wiley and Sons, 1991.

9. Ellis, Atkeson, Calhoun, 1982: Gidycz, Coble, Lathan Layman, (1993); Guthrie, Notgrass, 1992.

10. Frieze IH Browne A. Violence in marriage. In: Ohlin L, Tonry, M, eds. Family Violence: Crime and Justice, A Review of Research. Chicago, Ill: University of Chicago Press; 1989:163-218.

11. American Academy of Pediatrics, Committee on Adolescence. Sexual assault and the adolescent. Pediatrics. 1994;94(5):761-765.

12. Heise, L.L. Reproductive freedom and violence against women: where are the intersections? J Law Med Ethics. 1993;21(2):206-216.

235. FACTS ABOUT RAPE

➡ Women do not provoke sexual violence. No matter what the circumstances, it is never someone's fault if she/he is raped.

➡ Rape is a crime of violence—not passion

➡ All survivors react differently to rape

➡ Only a small number of rapes that occur are reported

➡ In over 80% of rapes, the victim knows the rapist

➡ Reported rape victims in Florida range in age from 2 months to 91 years

➡ It is very important that survivors be given the opportunity to make their own life decisions following an attack

➡ If someone you know is raped, it is imperative that you believe, support, and refrain from blaming him/her

➡ Sexual violence can affect many areas of your life and make you feel like you've lost control, even years after the assault. Healing takes time but you can feel okay again.

Source: Refuge House Facts About Rape Page, 1997. Internet address: http://fn3.freenet.tlh.fl.us/RefugeHouse/rapefacts.html

236. STEPS FOR PREVENTING SEXUAL ASSAULT OR RAPE

Often, this emotionally devastating crime can be decreased by following these suggestions:

➡ Believe that your body belongs to you. You don't have to do anything that you don't want to do with it. Only you can choose what you want.

➡ Set your limits and state them clearly. If sexual attention or advances are not wanted, say "NO" clearly and assertively, and repeatedly.

➡ If you are unsure of what you want, it is okay to say that. You also need to state clearly that, at least for the present time, this means "NO."

➡ Trust your instincts. The moment you feel uncomfortable, ACT. If saying that you want to stop does not stop the unwanted behavior, don't be afraid to make a scene. Protect yourself.

➡ If your initial "No" and other protests do not stop an unwanted advance, YELL for help, or get physically out of the situation

➡ Always walk in pairs at night

➡ If you jog at night, jog with a friend

➡ Stay away from darkened streets, alleys, buildings, and bushes

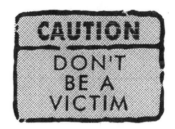

➡ Carry keys between a closed fist and use them to rake across an attacker's face. Remember, legal weapons such as mace, umbrellas, fingernail files, etc. can be turned against you.

➡ Walk confidently and on the side of the street facing traffic

➡ If at any time you feel in danger, don't be reluctant to scream and run. Carry a whistle or any other type of noisemaker.

➡ If you are being followed, go to the nearest populated place. If you are walking alone think ahead of the nearest place of assistance such as a friend's house or a public place.

➡ Always check the rear seat of your car before entering

➡ Always lock the doors of your home and car before leaving

➡ Park in well-lighted areas and don't accept rides from strangers

➡ Always let someone know where you are, where you will be, and when you'll be back

➡ If you are attacked, don't try to defeat the attacker, just get away as quickly as possible

➡ Usually a rapist expects a timid or passive reaction. Try yelling, hitting, biting, poking the eyes, or kicking to gain a chance to escape. Be realistic about your self-defense ability in order to prevent increased injury to yourself.

➡ If your life is clearly in danger, passive resistance may be advisable. Claiming to be sick, pregnant, or infected with a sexual transmitted disease may deter the attacker. Attempt to calm or discourage the rapist.

➡ Most important, remember to think and avoid situations that could compromise your safety

Source: SUNY Brockport Student Affairs. Internet address: http://cc.brockport.edu/~health-sr/ccrape.html

237. FACTS ABOUT DOMESTIC VIOLENCE

➡ Battering is the single major cause of injury to women, more than auto accidents, muggings, and rapes combined

➡ According to the F.B.I. statistics, a woman is beaten every 9 seconds

➡ 50 to 70 percent of husbands who batter their wives also batter their children

➡ Battered mothers indicate that 87 percent of their children witness the abuse

➡ 50 to 60 percent of abusers come from homes where they were abused or witnessed abuse

➡ Abuser use threats, intimidation, isolation, denial, economics and blaming the victim, as well as physical and sexual violence to control

➡ Domestic violence affects all socioeconomic, racial, class, and ethnic groups

Source: Refuge House Facts About Rape Page, 1997. Internet address: http://fn3.freenet.tlh.fl.us/RefugeHouse/rapefacts.html

238. SYMPTOMS OF DOMESTIC ABUSE

The following are symptoms of domestic abuse (misuse of power and control):

USING EMOTIONAL ABUSE

➡ Put-downs

➡ Name-calling

➡ Playing mind games

➡ Humiliation

➡ Attempting to make a person feel guilty

➡ Attempting to make a person feel as if he or she is "crazy"

USING MALE PRIVILEGE

➡ Treating a woman like a servant

➡ Making all the big decisions

➡ Acting like "Master of the Castle"

➡ Being the one to define men's and women's roles

USING ECONOMIC ABUSE

➡ Preventing a person from getting or keeping a job

➡ Making the person ask for money

➡ Giving a partner an allowance

➡ Taking a partner's money

➡ Not giving information or access to family income

USING COERCION AND THREATS

➡ Making or carrying out threats to do something to hurt a person

➡ Threatening to leave, commit suicide, to report a person to welfare

➡ Making a person drop charges

➡ Making a person do illegal things

USING INTIMIDATION

➡ Scaring someone by using looks, gestures, or actions

➡ Smashing things

➡ Abusing pets

➡ Displaying weapons

USING CHILDREN

➡ Trying to make a partner feel guilty about the children

➡ Using the children to relay messages

➡ Using visitation to harass partner

➡ Threatening to take the children away

USING ISOLATION

➡ Controlling what a person does, who a person sees and talks to, what a person reads, and where a person goes

➡ Limiting a person's outside involvement

➡ Using jealousy to justify actions

MINIMIZING, DENYING, BLAMING

➡ Making light of the abuse and not taking a partner's concerns seriously

➡ Saying the abuse didn't happen

➡ Shifting responsibility for abusive behavior

➡ Saying the partner caused the abuse

Adapted from: Domestic Abuse. Metro Nashville Police Department. 1997. Internet address: http://www.telalink.net/~police/abuse/index.html

239. RECOGNIZING THE BATTERER

The following are signs of a batterer:

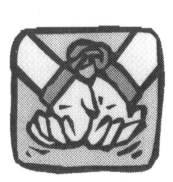

1. A batterer is jealous.
2. A batterer blames others for his/her faults.
3. A batterer blames circumstances for existing problems.
4. A batterer demonstrates unpredictable behavior.
5. A batterer belittles his/her partner verbally.
6. A batterer cannot control anger or personal rage.
7. A batterer always asks for a second chance.
8. A batterer says he/she will change—that he/she won't do it again.
9. A batterer may have been an abused child, or witnessed parental abuse and violence.
10. A batterer plays on the partner's guilt. (If you loved me you'd...)
11. A batterers' behavior often becomes worse when drugs and alcohol are used.
12. A batterer is close-minded. His/Her way is the only way.
13. A batterer may seem charming, gregarious, gentle to non-family members.
14. A batterer abuses his/her children.

Source: Signs of the Batterer, 1997. Internet address: http://www.getnet.com/~pvi/women/signs.html

240. "SWEET BABY" SYNDROMES

These are methods a male batterer may use in order to "come back":

HONEYMOON SYNDROME

➡ Also known as "Hearts and Flowers"—any bribe that will get her to return to him

SUPER DAD SYNDROME

➡ He tells her that he will be a great dad if she returns. This is effective especially if he has neglected the children in the past.

REVIVAL SYNDROME

➡ He tells her that he has accepted Christ into his life. He puts the responsibility for his battering on God. He tells her he has been to church every Sunday since she left.

SOBRIETY SYNDROME

➡ He tells her that he has stopped drinking, and she believes that if he stops drinking, he will stop beating her. Drinking does not cause beating; if it did, batterers would beat strangers on the street.

COUNSELING SYNDROME

➡ He tells her that he has gone to counseling and that he won't do it anymore. Long term counseling is needed, and less than 1% voluntarily go into counseling.

Adapted from: Domestic Abuse. Metro Nashville Police Department, 1997.
Internet address: http://www.telalink.net/~police/abuse/index.html

241.   COMMON CHARACTERISTICS OF THE BATTERER

A batterer may:

➡ have low self-esteem

➡ believe all the myths about battering relationships

➡ be a traditionalist , believing in male supremacy and the stereotyped masculine sex role in the family

➡ blame others for his/her actions

➡ be pathologically jealous

➡ present a dual personality

➡ have severe stress reactions during which he/she uses drinking and battering to cope

➡ frequently use sex as an act of aggression to enhance his self-esteem

➡ not believe that violent behavior should have negative consequences

Adapted from: Domestic Abuse, 1997. Metro Nashville Police Department.
Internet address: http://www.telalink.net/~police/abuse/index.html
Walker, Lenore, *The Battered Woman.*

242.   COMMON CHARACTERISTICS OF BATTERED WOMEN

A battered woman may

➡ have low self-esteem

➡ believe all the myths about battering relationships

➡ be a traditionalist about the home

➡ strongly believe in family unity and the prescribed feminine sex-role stereotype

➡ accept responsibility for the batterer's actions

➡ suffer from guilt, yet deny the terror and anger she feels

➡ have severe stress reactions with psychological and physiological complaints

➡ use sex as a way to establish intimacy

➡ believe that no one will be able to help her resolve her predicament

Adapted from: Domestic Abuse. Metro Nashville Police Department 1997.
Internet address: http://www.telalink.net/~police/abuse/index.html

243. HOTLINE NUMBERS

The following is a list of hotlines and other contact numbers for battered women:

NATIONAL HOTLINE   1-800-799-SAFE

STATE TOLL FREE HOTLINES

Arkansas	1-800-332-4443
Indiana	1-800-334-7233
L.A. County	1-800-978-3600
Michigan	1-800-99-NO ABUSE or 1-800-996-6228
Montana	1-800-655-7867 (24 hours)
Nevada	1-800-992-5757
New Hampshire	1-800-852-3311
New Jersey	1-800-572-7233
New York	1-800-942-6906 (English)
New York	1-800-942-6908 (Spanish)
North Dakota	1-800-472-2911
Oklahoma	1-800-522-7233
Pennsylvania (eastern)	1-800-642-3150
Texarkana Area	1-800-876-4808 or local calls 903-793-help
Washington	1-800-562-6025
Wisconsin	1-800-333-7233
Wyoming	(SAFV Task Force of Uinta County) 307-789-7315 or 800-445-7233

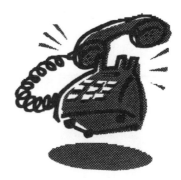

FOR A LISTING OF EVERY DOMESTIC VIOLENCE COALITION CONTACT:

National Resource Center on Domestic Violence, 1-800-537-2238.

The following is a list of national hotlines for abused, missing, runaway or exploited children:

800-I-AM-LOST Child Find Hotline (parents reporting lost children) (800-426-5678)

800-4-A-CHILD Child Help USA (for victims, offenders, and parents) (800-422-4453)

800-999-9999 Covenant House Hotline (for problem teens and runaways)

800-A-WAY-OUT (hotline for parents considering abducting their children)

800-843-5678 National Center for Missing and Exploited Children

800-231-6946 National Runaway Hotline

800-442-HOPE National Youth Crisis Hotline   (800-442-4673)

800-782-SEEK Operation Lookout, National Center for Missing Youth (800-782-7335) (for missing child emergencies and sightings)

800-HIT-HOME Youth Crisis Hotline (800-448-4663) (reporting child abuse and help for runaways)

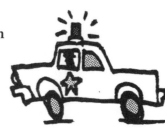

Source: Internet: http://www.iquest.net/~gtemp/htlines.htm 1997.

244. PUBLIC HEALTH SERVICE AGENCIES AND SOURCES OF INFORMATION

OFFICE ON WOMEN'S HEALTH
US Public Health Service
Humphrey Building, Room 730B
200 Independence Ave, SW
Washington, DC 20201
(202) 690-7650
Internet Address: http://www.4woman.org

THE AGENCY FOR HEALTH CARE POLICY AND RESEARCH (AHCPR)

Conducts research on the quality, effectiveness, and appropriateness of health care and access to health care services. Currently conducting a study that addresses the early identification of victims of domestic violence.

THE CENTERS FOR DISEASE CONTROL AND PREVENTION (CDC)
NATIONAL CENTER FOR INJURY PREVENTION AND CONTROL (NCIPC)
4770 Buford Highway, NE, MS: F-36
Atlanta, GA 30341-3724
(404) 488-4690

Operates a comprehensive program to prevent violence that occurs in the context of families and intimate relationships

THE HEALTH RESOURCES AND SERVICES ADMINISTRATION (HRSA)

Has leadership responsibility for general health service and resource issues relating to access, equity, quality, and cost of care. The reduction of domestic violence is of critical concern to HRSA.

THE INDIAN HEALTH SERVICE (IHS)

Provides health care services and assistance to American Indian and Alaskan Native women.

THE NATIONAL INSTITUTES OF HEALTH (NIH)
Office of Extramural Research
Building 15K, Room 180 of Health
15 North Drive
Bethesda, MD 20892-2668
(301) 496-4406

Provides scientific leadership and supports scientific research on women's health.

THE SUBSTANCE ABUSE AND MENTAL HEALTH SERVICES ADMINISTRATION (SAMHSA)
Office for Women's Services
5600 Fishers Lane, Parklawn Bldg.
Room 13-99
Rockville, MD 20857
(301) 443-5184

Recognizes violence as a priority for its programs and has embarked on a variety of activities that address violence against women.

THE ADMINISTRATION FOR CHILDREN AND FAMILIES (ACF)
Aerospace Center Building
370 L'Enfant Promenade, SW, Room 610
Washington, DC 20447
(202) 401-9200

Within the Department of Health and Human Services (DHHS); supports state and local programs to prevent family violence and provide temporary shelter for women and children.

SECTION 13

SUBSTANCE ABUSE

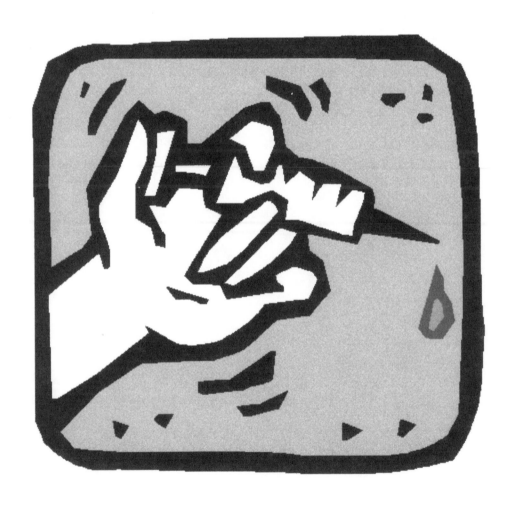

245. FACTORS THAT DISCOURAGE DRUG USE

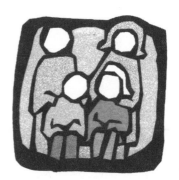

➠ Being reared in a loving, functional family

➠ Being involved in school activities

➠ Having positive self-esteem

➠ Having clearly defined goals and plans to reach them

➠ Having friends who do not use drugs

➠ Feeling a sense of accomplishment

➠ Having positive adult role models

➠ Having a healthy attitude concerning competition

➠ Being committed to following society's rules

➠ Having a plan to cope with life stressors

246. FACTORS THAT ENCOURAGE DRUG USE

➠ Being reared in a dysfunctional family

➠ Having negative self-esteem

➠ Being unable to resist peer pressure

➠ Having difficulty mastering developmental tasks. Being economically disadvantaged

➠ Having a genetic background with a predisposition towards chemical dependency

➠ Suffering from depression

➠ Experiencing excessive pressure to succeed

➠ Having difficulty achieving success in school

➠ Suffering from attention deficit-hyperactive disorder

➠ Suffering from immature character disorder

➠ Having borderline personality tendencies

247. METHODS OF DRUG ADMINISTRATION

ABSORPTION   Applying the drug to the body so that it may be absorbed into the body through one of the following methods:

      Transdermal administration—through the skin surface
      Sublingual administration—under the tongue
      Buccal administration—between the cheek and gum.

BAGGING   Spraying an aerosol or placing the solvent into a bag, placing the bag over the mouth and nose, and inhaling deeply.

HUFFING   Sniffing the vapors from a cloth soaked with the solvent.

INHALATION   Inhaling or breathing of the vapors from the substance.

INJECTION   Injecting a drug into the body through one of the following methods:

      Subcutaneous administration—just below the skin
      Intramuscular—administration into the muscle
      Intravenous—administration (IV) directly into the bloodstream.

ORAL INGESTION   Taking the drug by mouth; the most common method.

SNORTING   Sniffing the drug through the nostrils.

248. FACTORS THAT INFLUENCE DRUG REACTIONS

BLOOD-BRAIN BARRIER   Most of the drugs of abuse affect the brain cells. Fat-insoluble drugs have difficulty passing through the barrier. Fat-soluble drugs have less difficulty passing through the capillary walls.

DOSAGE   The amount or quantity of a drug that is administered within a specified time period can produce dose-related effects.

PLATEAUING EFFECT   In some cases, taking more of a drug beyond a certain amount or dosage will not increase the intensity of its effects.

DRUG INTERACTIONS   When taking more than one drug at a time, there is a risk of adverse drug effects in the action of one drug on another.

USER EXPECTATIONS   The user's beliefs about the drug can affect the user's reaction to that drug.

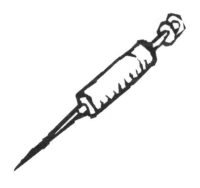

249. CONTROLLED SUBSTANCES—USES AND EFFECTS

Controlled Substances - *Uses &*

DRUGS/ CSA SCHEDULES		TRADE OR OTHER NAMES	MEDICAL USES	DEPENDENCE Physical
NARCOTICS				
Opium	II III V	Dover's Powder, Paregoric Parepectolin	Analgesic, antidiarrheal	High
Morphine	II III	Morphine, MS-Contin, Roxanol, Roxanol-SR	Analgesic, antitussive	High
Codeine	II III V	Tylenol w/Codeine, Empirin w/Codeine Robitussan A-C, Fiorinal w/Codeine	Analgesic, antitussive	Moderate
Heroin	I	Diacetylmorphine, Horse, Smack	None	High
Hydromorphone	II	Dilaudid	Analgesic	High
Meperidine (Pethidine)	II	Demerol, Mepergan	Analgesic	High
Methadone	II	Dolophine, Methadone, Methadose	Analgesic	High
Other Narcotics I II III IV V		Numorphan, Percodan, Percocet, Tylox, Tussionex, Fentanyl, Darvon, Lomotil, Talwin[2]	Analgesic, antidiarrheal, antitussive	High-Low
DEPRESSANTS				
Chloral Hydrate	IV	Noctec	Hypnotic	Moderate
Barbiturates	II III IV	Amytal, Butisol, Fiorinal, Lotusate, Nembutal, Seconal, Tuinal, Phenobarbital	Anesthetic, anticonvulsant, sedative, hypnotic, veterinary euthanasia agent	High-Mod.
Benzodiazepines	IV	Ativan, Dalmane, Diazepam, Librium, Xanax, Serax, Valium Tranxexe, Verstran, Versed, Halcion, Paxipam, Restoril	Antianxiety, anticonvulsant, sedative, hypnotic	Low
Methaqualone	I	Quaalude	Sedative, hypnotic	High
Glutethimide	III	Doriden	Sedative, hypnotic	High
Other Depressants	III IV	Equanil, Miltown, Noludar, Placidyl, Valmid	Antianxiety, sedative, hypnotic	Moderate
STIMULANTS				
Cocaine[1]	II	Coke, Flake, Snow, Crack	Local anesthetic	Possible
Amphetamines	II	Biphetamine, Delcobese, Desoxyn, Dexedrine, Obetrol	Attention deficit disorders, narcolepsy, weight control	Possible
Phenmetrazine	II	Preludin	Weight control	Possible
Methylphenidate	II	Ritalin	Attention deficit disorders, narcolepsy	Possible
Other Stimulants	III IV	Adipex, Cylert, Didrex, Ionamin, Melfiat, Plegine, Sanorex, Tenuate, Tepanil, Prelu-2	Weight Control	Possible
HALLUCINOGENS				
LSD	I	Acid, Microdot	None	None
Mescaline and Peyote	I	Mexc, Buttons, Cactus	None	None
Amphetamine Variants	I	2,5-DMA, PMA, STP, MDA, MDMA, TMA, DOM, DOB	None	Unknown
Phencyclidine	II	PCP, Angel Dust, Hog	None	Unknown
Phencyclidine Analogues	I	PCE, PCPy, TCP	None	Unknown
Other Hallucinogens	I	Bufotenine, Ibogaine, DMT, DET, Psilocybin, Psilocyn	None	None
CANNABIS				
Marijuana	I	Pot, Acapulco Gold, Grass, Reefer, Sinsemilla, Thai Sticks	None	Unknown
Tetrahydrocannabinol	I II	THC, Marinol	Cancer chemotherapy antinauseant	Unknown
Hashish	I	Hash	None	Unknown
Hashish Oil	I	Hash Oil	None	Unknown

[1] Designated a narcotic under the CSA.   [2] Not designated a narcotic under the CSA.

(continued)

249. CONTROLLED SUBSTANCES—USES AND EFFECTS *(continued)*

Effects

DEPENDENCE Psychological	TOLERANCE	DURATION (Hours)	USUAL METHODS OF ADMINISTRATION	POSSIBLE EFFECTS	EFFECTS OF OVERDOSE	WITHDRAWAL SYNDROME
High	Yes	3-6	Oral, smoked	Euphoria, drowsiness, respiratory depression, constricted pupils, nausea	Slow and shallow breathing, clammy skin, convulsions, coma, possible death	Watery eyes, runny nose, yawning, loss of appetite, irritability, tremors, panic, cramps, nausea, chills and sweating
High	Yes	3-6	Oral, smoked, injected			
Moderate	Yes	3-6	Oral, injected			
High	Yes	3-6	Injected, sniffed, smoked			
High	Yes	3-6	Oral, injected			
High	Yes	3-6	Oral, injected			
High-Low	Yes	12-24	Oral, injected			
High-Low	Yes	Variable	Oral, injected			
Moderate	Yes	5-8	Oral	Slurred speech, disorientation, drunken behavior without odor of alcohol	Shallow respiration, clammy skin, dilated pupils, weak and rapid pulse, coma, possible death	Anxiety, insomnia, tremors, delirium, convulsions, possible death
High-Mod.	Yes	1-16	Oral			
Low	Yes	4-8	Oral			
High	Yes	4-8	Oral			
Moderate	Yes	4-8	Oral			
Moderate	Yes	4-8	Oral			
High	Yes	1-2	Sniffed, smoked, injected	Increased alertness, excitation, euphoria, increased pulse rate & blood pressure, insomnia, loss of appetite	Agitation, increase in body temperature, hallucinations, convulsions, possible death	Apathy, long periods of sleep, irritability, depression, disorientation
High	Yes	2-4	Oral, injected			
High	Yes	2-4	Oral, injected			
Moderate	Yes	2-4	Oral, injected			
High	Yes	2-4	Oral, injected			
Unknown	Yes	8-12	Oral	Illusions and hallucinations, poor perception of time and distance	Longer, more intense "trip" episodes, psychosis, possible death	Withdrawal syndrome not reported
Unknown	Yes	8-12	Oral			
Unknown	Yes	Variable	Oral, injected			
High	Yes	Days	Smoked, oral, injected			
High	Yes	Days	Smoked, oral, injected			
Unknown	Possible	Variable	Smoked, oral, injected, sniffed			
Moderate	Yes	2-4	Smoked, oral	Euphoria, relaxed inhibitions, increased appetite, disoriented behavior	Fatigue, paranoia, possible psychosis	Insomnia, hyperactivity, and decreased appetite occasionally reported
Moderate	Yes	2-4	Smoked, oral			
Moderate	Yes	2-4	Smoked, oral			
Moderate	Yes	2-4	Smoked, oral			

Source: U.S. Department of Justice, Drug Enforcement Administration, *Controlled Substances: Use, Abuse, and Effects.*

250. SOME SOURCES OF CAFFEINE

➡ Coffee
➡ Tea
➡ Soda
➡ Chocolate
➡ Chocolate-flavored products
➡ Some prescription drugs

➡ Allergy remedies
➡ Cold remedies
➡ Alertness pills
➡ Analgesic compounds
➡ Diuretics
➡ Weight control aids

251. CAFFEINE CONTENT OF SOME BEVERAGES AND OVER-THE-COUNTER DRUGS

Average amount of caffeine in a 7-ounce cup of coffee or tea:

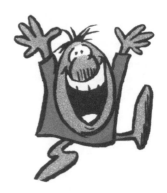

Coffee	Milligrams
Automatic drip	115-175
Brewed	80-135
Espresso (one 1.5-2 oz. serving)	100
Instant	65-100
Decaffeinated, brewed	3-4
Decaffeinated, instant	2-3

Tea	
Iced (12 oz)	70
Imported, brewed	60
U.S., brewed	40
Instant	30

Average amount of caffeine in a 12-ounce soft-drink can, according to the National Soft Drink Association (in rounded figures):

Soda	
Jolt	71
Sugar-Free Mr. Pibb	59
Mountain Dew	55
Diet Mountain Dew	55
Mellow Yellow	53

Soda (cont'd)

Soda (cont'd)	Milligrams
Tab	47
Coca-Cola	46
Diet Cola	46
Shasta Cola	44
Shasta Diet Cola	44
Shasta Cherry Cola	44
Mr. Pibb	41
Dr. Pepper	40
Pepsi Cola	37
RC Cola	36
Diet RC	36
Canada Dry Cola	36
Diet Pepsi	35
Diet Rite Cola	30
Canada Dry Diet Cola	1
Ginger Ale	0
Pepsi Free	0
7 Up	0

Chocolate

Chocolate	
Drink made from cocoa (6 oz.)	10
Baking chocolate (1 oz.)	35
Milk chocolate (1 oz.)	6

Nonprescription drugs, one tablet

Nonprescription drugs, one tablet	
Anacin	32
Aspirin	0
Dexatrim	200
Excedrin	65
Midol	32
NoDoz	100

Note: Although milligrams are stated in exact amounts, we remind readers that beverage manufacturers may change the content and proportions at any time. Our research through content lists from 1987 to the present showed many variations. In fact, most brands have higher caffeine content than earlier, but many have also introduced caffeine-free variations to the market.

252. COMMON TYPES OF INHALANTS AND THEIR EFFECTS

Household Chemicals	Effects of Household Chemicals
Deodorants and Antiperspirants	Altered states of consciousness
Dry-Cleaning Fluids	Changes in behaviors
Fingernail Polish Remover	Seizures and sudden death
Furniture Polish and Shoe Polish	Increased accidents
Gas Jets in School Science Labs	Kidney and liver failure
Gasoline and Transmission Fluids	Heart muscle damage
Glues and Contact Cements	Skeletal muscle weakness
Hair Sprays	Irritation in directly exposed areas
Lighter Fluid and Marker Fluids	Brain and nerve damage
Liquid Waxes and Window Cleaners	Bone marrow suppression
Over-the-Counter Nasal Inhalants	Leukemia
Paper Correction Fluid	Lead poisoning
Spray Paints and Paint Thinners	Fetal and infant abnormalities

Nitrite Inhalants	Effects of Nitrite Inhalants
Amyl Nitrite (Poppers, Snappers)	Dizziness and fainting
Butyl Nitrite	Rapid pulse
Isobutyl Nitrite	Feelings of warmth
	Heat loss and subsequent chill
	Throbbing sensations
	Perspiration
	Flushing of the face
	Headache and nausea

Nitrous Oxide	Effects of Nitrous Oxide
(Laughing Gas)	Nausea
	Lightheadedness
	Visual hallucinations
	Detachment from reality
	Loss of motivation
	Reduced inhibitions
	Loss of consciousness
	Loss of motor control
	Freezing of mouth and lips
	Respiratory depression
	Kidney and liver disease
	Depressed bone marrow function
	Spontaneous miscarriage
	Disturbances in heart rhythm

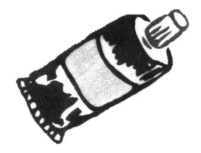

253. SOURCES OF STEROIDS AND REASONS FOR THEIR USE

SOURCES OF STEROIDS

➠ Produced overseas, smuggled into the United States, and sold through the black market
➠ Produced in "underground" laboratories in the United States
➠ Produced by U.S. pharmaceutical companies, find their way into the black market

REASONS FOR STEROID USE

➠ To enhance physical appearance
➠ To achieve positive self-esteem
➠ To enhance athletic performance
➠ To enhance muscular strength

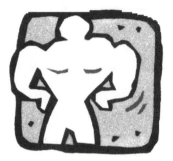

254. MEDICAL USES AND EFFECTS OF STEROIDS

STEROIDS ARE USED MEDICALLY TO TREAT

➠ Certain types of anemia
➠ Some breast cancers
➠ Osteoporosis
➠ Severe burns
➠ Testosterone deficiency
➠ Endometriosis

EFFECTS OF STEROID USE

➠ Acne
➠ Jaundice
➠ Trembling
➠ Swelling of feet or ankles
➠ Bad breath
➠ Reduction in "good cholesterol"
➠ High blood pressure
➠ Liver damage and cancers
➠ Aching joints
➠ Increased injury to tendons

EFFECTS ON MALES

➠ Shrinking of the testicles
➠ Reduced sperm count
➠ Impotence
➠ Baldness
➠ Difficulty or pain in urinating
➠ Development of breasts
➠ Enlarged prostate

EFFECTS ON FEMALES

➠ Growth of facial hair
➠ Cessation of the menstrual cycle
➠ Enlargement of the clitoris
➠ Deepened voice
➠ Breast reduction

255. MOST-ABUSED ALCOHOLIC BEVERAGES

BEER AND ALE

➟ Made by fermentation of grains and malt. Hops may be added for distinctive flavor. Most contain 4–7% alcohol.

WINE (CHAMPAGNE, RED, WHITE, ETC.)

➟ Made by fermentation of grapes or other fruit. Regular wine contains 9–14% alcohol. (Dessert wines, such as port and sherry, contain 18–21% alcohol.)

HARD LIQUOR (WHISKEY, GIN, VODKA, RUM, ETC.)

➟ Made by distillation of a fermented brew of grain, fruit, or molasses. Contains 40–50% alcohol (80–100 proof).

256.   PHYSICAL EFFECTS OF ALCOHOL USE

ALCOHOL USE CAN CAUSE:

➟ Puffiness of face
➟ Depression of body systems
➟ Shallow respiration
➟ Cold, clammy skin
➟ Irregular heartbeat
➟ Dehydration

➟ Redness of eyes
➟ Disorientation
➟ Nausea
➟ Blurred vision
➟ High blood pressure

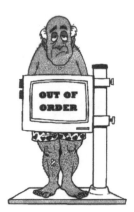

FREQUENT USE CAN LEAD TO:

➟ Cirrhosis of liver
➟ Brain disorders
➟ Malnutrition
➟ Cancer of the stomach
➟ Heart disease
➟ Birth defects

➟ Pancreatitis
➟ Vitamin deficiencies
➟ Cancer of the mouth
➟ Cancer of the liver
➟ Ulcers
➟ DT's (delirium tremens)

257. EFFECTS OF BLOOD ALCOHOL CONCENTRATION

Effects of alcohol consumed in a two-hour period on a 100-pound person:

UP TO 0.05 PERCENT (1–2 DRINKS)

➡ The user will generally experience some recognizable sensations, including lightheaded-ness, a sense of relaxation and well-being, an elevation of mood, some loss of coordina-tion, and slower reaction time. There may also be a release of some personal inhibitions, so that the drinker may say or do things that are not in his or her normal behavioral pattern.

BETWEEN 0.06 AND 0.10 PERCENT (3–4 DRINKS)

➡ The user will suffer a loss of some motor coordination, a greater delay in reaction time, and some impairment of judgment and perception. Emotions and inhibitions become relaxed.

BETWEEN 0.10 AND 0.20 PERCENT (5–6 DRINKS)

➡ There is significant impairment of motor coordination and reaction time. The drinker may stagger slightly, fumble objects, and have some trouble saying even familiar words. Unpredictable emotional behavior may be exhibited.

AT 0.30 PERCENT (7–8 DRINKS)

➡ The drinker will be severely intoxicated, and both physically and psychologically inca-pacitated. He or she will experience double vision, hearing impairment, and difficulty with depth perception.

AT 0.40 PERCENT (9–10 DRINKS)

➡ BAC concentrations at this level lead to coma and are lethal for about 50 percent of the drinkers. The drinker's nervous system shuts down and he or she may experience vom-iting or uncontrolled urination.

AT 0.50 PERCENT (MORE THAN 10 DRINKS)

➡ Coma may occur, brain is unable to control body temper-ature and breathing. BAC concentrations at this level would cause suffocation and death for 99 percent of the drinkers.

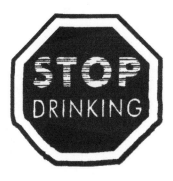

258. ALCOHOL IMPAIRMENT CHARTS

Men

Approximate Blood Alcohol Percentage

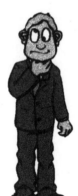

Never Drink and Drive!

Drinks	Body Weight in Pounds								
	100	120	140	160	180	200	220	240	
1	.04	.03	.03	.02	.02	.02	.02	.02	Impairment Begins
2	.08	.06	.05	.05	.04	.04	.03	.03	Driving Skills
3	.11	.09	.08	.07	.06	.06	.05	.05	Significantly Affected
4	.15	.12	.11	.09	.08	.08	.07	.06	
5	.19	.16	.13	.12	.11	.09	.09	.08	Possible Criminal
6	.23	.19	.16	.14	.13	.11	.10	.09	Penalties
7	.26	.22	.19	.16	.15	.13	.12	.11	Legally
8	.30	.25	.21	.19	.17	.15	.14	.13	Intoxicated
9	.34	.28	.24	.21	.19	.17	.15	.14	Criminal
10	.38	.31	.27	.23	.21	.19	.17	.16	Penalties

Subtract .01% for each 40 minutes of drinking.
One drink is 1.25 oz. of 80 proof liquor, 12 oz. of beer, or 5 oz. of table wine.

Women

Approximate Blood Alcohol Percentage

Drinks	Body Weight in Pounds								
	90	100	120	140	160	180	200	220	240
1	.05	.05	.04	.03	.03	.03	.02	.02	.02
2	.10	.09	.08	.07	.06	.05	.05	.04	.04
3	.15	.14	.11	.10	.09	.08	.07	.06	.06
4	.20	.18	.15	.13	.11	.10	.09	.08	.08
5	.25	.23	.19	.16	.14	.13	.11	.10	.09
6	.30	.27	.23	.19	.17	.15	.14	.12	.11
7	.35	.32	.27	.23	.20	.18	.16	.14	.13
8	.40	.36	.30	.26	.23	.20	.18	.17	.15
9	.45	.41	.34	.29	.26	.23	.20	.19	.17
10	.51	.45	.38	.32	.28	.25	.23	.21	.19

Impairment labels (Women):
- 1 — Impairment Begins
- 2–3 — Driving Skills Significantly Affected
- 4–5 — Possible Criminal Penalties
- 6–7 — Legally Intoxicated
- 8–10 — Criminal Penalties

Subtract .01% for each 40 minutes of drinking.
One drink is 1.25 oz. of 80 proof liquor, 12 oz. of beer, or 5 oz. of table wine.

Source: Pennsylvania Liquor Control Board. Reprinted with permission.

259. FACTORS THAT CAN INFLUENCE THE EFFECTS OF ALCOHOL

PRESENCE OF FOOD IN STOMACH
Dilutes the alcohol and extends the time it takes for alcohol to pass into the small intestine.

BODY SIZE
The higher a person's body weight, the more alcohol it will take to become intoxicated.

BODY COMPOSITION
Body fat does not absorb alcohol as quickly as lean body tissue.

GENDER
Females have a higher proportion of body fat than males, which affects the absorption rate of alcohol. Female hormones also seem to make them more sensitive to the effects of alcohol.

AGE
The older a person, the higher the incidence for high blood-alcohol concentrations due to the lower volumes of body fluids.

260. CHARACTERISTICS OF ALCOHOLISM

GREATER TOLERANCE
Drinks more and more for the same effect. Eventually, has trouble stopping drinking once he or she starts.

BLACKOUTS
Has no recall of things that were said or done while drinking.

DENIAL
Tries to deny alcohol is a problem. May even abstain for a while to "prove" that he or she is not addicted.

PERSONALITY CHANGES
May be tense, irritable, moody. May isolate self and lose ambition, causing problems at home, school or work.

OBVIOUS UN-CONTROLLED DRINKING
Continues to drink despite painful and destructive effects on health, career, and personal relationships.

OTHER INDICATIONS
May gulp drinks, sneak drinks, drink in the morning or when alone, or suffer malnutrition and delirium tremens.

261. COMMON TREATMENTS FOR ALCOHOLISM

MEDICAL TREATMENT

➡ Detoxification—physical withdrawal from alcohol

➡ Restriction from addicting substances

➡ Teaching the disease model of addiction

➡ Treatment of associated psychiatric problems

➡ Periodic unscheduled alcohol blood tests

➡ Encouragement of exercise

CHEMICAL TREATMENT

➡ Chlordiazepoxide-to treat alcohol withdrawal symptoms

➡ Multivitamins-to prevent the progression of alcohol withdrawal symptoms

➡ Disulfiram (Antabuse)-causes a toxic reaction to alcohol that assists in the prevention of relapses

➡ Antidepressant drugs-to prevent symptoms of depression

➡ Antipsychotic drugs-for use in cases where the alcoholic suffers from alcohol induced hallucinations

PSYCHOSOCIAL TREATMENT

➡ Psychotherapy-to assist the alcoholic in confronting his or her denial and addiction

➡ Alcoholics Anonymous (AA)-provides members with acceptance, understanding, forgiveness, confrontation, and a means for positive identification

➡ Residential Care and Halfway House-provides emotional support, counseling, and progressive entry into society

➡ Behavior Therapy-teaches the alcoholic other ways to reduce anxiety

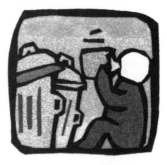

262. FACTORS THAT AFFECT ALCOHOL USE BY YOUTH

➠ Alcohol is readily available to youth

➠ Being drunk is an expectation in most adolescent drinking situations

➠ Peer group influence is strongly evident

➠ Young drinkers tend to obtain their alcohol from parents

➠ Young drinkers tend to consume the alcohol at home

➠ Students who drink alcohol regularly are more likely to have someone close to them who also drinks alcohol

➠ Students tend to regard drinking as a legitimate pastime. Students tend to regard drinking as an essential aspect of leisure and entertainment.

➠ Students lack knowledge about alcohol

➠ Students do not know how to monitor their intake to prevent intoxication

➠ Students lack knowledge of the properties and effects of alcohol. Students lack knowledge as to how alcohol is metabolized.

➠ Alcohol is readily available at most social functions

MOST COMMON REASONS FOR TEENAGE DRINKING:

➠ Peer influence

➠ Curiosity

➠ Enjoyment

➠ Having fun

➠ Relaxation

➠ Gaining confidence

➠ Forgetting problems

➠ Availability

➠ Boredom

➠ Rebellion

263. COMMON CHARACTERISTICS OF YOUNG SMOKERS

➡ Have more spendable income than teenagers who have never smoked

➡ Have a parent who smokes

➡ Have an older sibling who smokes

➡ Associates with other young smokers

➡ Are left at home alone without supervision for ten or more hours per week

➡ Know more people who use chewing tobacco, snuff, marijuana, crack, and cocaine than nonsmokers

➡ Know more people who are sexually active than nonsmokers

➡ Report liking school less than nonsmokers

➡ Do less well in school than nonsmokers

➡ Perceive what they learn in school as being less useful to them later in life than do nonsmokers

➡ Absent from school more often than nonsmokers

➡ Cut school more often than nonsmokers

➡ Less likely than nonsmokers to attend religious services

➡ More likely than nonsmokers to:
   Feel tired
   Have trouble sleeping
   Be sad or depressed
   Feel hopeless, tense, or worried
   Be involved in risky behaviors

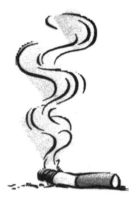

264. CHEMICAL COMPONENTS OF TOBACCO SMOKE

The estimated number of chemical compounds in tobacco smoke exceeds 4,000. Tar is a sticky, dark mixture of at least 3,500 of these chemicals in the cigarette smoke. Some of the chemicals are:

Nicotine	Ammonia
Cotinine	Hydrogen cyanide
Methane	Oxygen
Benzene	Carbon monoxide
Nitrogen	Carbon dioxide
Toluene	Formaldehyde

265. EFFECTS OF TOBACCO USE

Stained teeth
Smoker's breath
Dulled sense of taste
Shortness of breath
Stained fingers
Increased infant mortality
Thickening of artery walls
Formation of blood clots
Angina
Emphysema
Stomach cancer
Pancreatic cancer
Esophageal cancer
Laryngeal cancer
Constriction of small blood vessels

Atherosclerotic peripheral vascular disease
Chronic obstructive pulmonary disease
Unsuccessful pregnancy
Intrauterine growth retardation
Low birth weight, high-risk babies
"Tobacco jitters"
Reduction of lung efficiency
Chronic bronchitis
Coronary disease
Peptic ulcer disease
Kidney cancer
Bladder cancer
Oral cancers
Lung cancer
Increased susceptibility to minor ailments

EFFECTS OF SMOKING ON THE GROWING CHILD:

Impaired intellectual growth
Impaired physical growth
Higher incidence of asthma
Higher incidence of respiratory problems
Increased risk for pneumonia
Increased risk for bronchitis

Increased risk for ear infections
Behavioral problems:
    Lack of self-control
    Irritability
    Disinterest
    Hyperactivity

EFFECTS OF TOBACCO SMOKE ON NONSMOKERS:

Asthma
Eye irritation
Throat irritation
Airway irritation
Lung cancer
Chronic obstructive pulmonary disease
Lower respiratory tract infections
Middle ear infections in children
Interferes with developing lungs of growing children

EFFECTS OF SMOKELESS TOBACCO USE:

Leukoplakia (white patches on tongue and gums—sometimes precancerous)
Oral cancer
Tooth decay and loss
Gum recession
Abrasions of tooth enamel
Bad breath

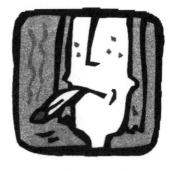

266. METHODS AND PROGRAMS TO QUIT SMOKING

ACUPUNCTURE   Use of needles or staplelike attachments in the ear or nose to relieve withdrawal symptoms.

AVERSIVE TECHNIQUES   Use of aversive stimuli such as electric shock, imagery, rapid smoking, and smoke holding to promote smoking behavior change.

COMMERCIAL PROGRAMS   "SmokEnders," "Smoke Stoppers," "Smokeless," and others offer classes and programs to assist in the cessation of smoking for a fee.

CONTINGENCY CONTRACTING   Contracts are established with the smoker that employ monetary rewards for not smoking and monetary punishments for smoking.

HYPNOSIS   Hypnosis is used to increase personal motivation to stop smoking by posthypnotically suggesting a link between smoking and unpleasant experiences.

NITOCINE-CONTAINING GUM   Use of nicotine gum to help alleviate such withdrawal symptoms as irritability, anxiety, problems in concentration, restlessness, and hunger.

NICOTINE FADING   Progressive reduction of nicotine intake by switching to brands with less nicotine and gradually decreasing the number of cigarettes smoked.

NICOTINE TRANSDERMAL PATCH   Use of a skin patch to deliver a constant level of nicotine in order to reduce withdrawal symptoms.

NONPHARMACOLOGIC CESSATION AIDS   Filter systems, smokeless cigarettes, self-help books, audiotapes, and videos are produced to assist in reducing or quitting smoking.

RELAXATION TRAINING   Provides smokers with a means other than smoking for coping with stress and negative emotions.

VOLUNTARY HEALTH AGENCY CESSATION PROGRAMS   Agencies such as the American Lung Association, American Cancer Society, and the National Cancer Institute offer programs to assist in the cessation of smoking.

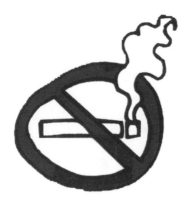

267. COMMON SIGNS OF DRUG MISUSE

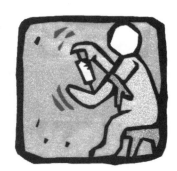

➠ Changes in attendance at work or school

➠ Changes from normal capabilities (work habits, efficiency, etc.)

➠ Poor physical appearance, including inattention to dress, personal hygiene, and eating habits

➠ Wearing sunglasses constantly at inappropriate times (indoors or at night, for example) to hide dilated or constricted pupils, to compensate for the eye's inability to adjust to sunlight, and to hide bloodshot eyes

➠ Unusual efforts made to cover arms in order to hide needle marks

➠ Association with known drug users

➠ Stealing items that can be easily sold for cash to support drug habit

268. COMMON DRUG TREATMENT APPROACHES

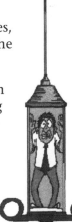

DETOXIFICATION

Stabilization of the heavy alcohol or other drug user until his or her body is free of the addicting drug.

INPATIENT HOSPITAL PROGRAMS

Residential programs, in hospitals or in other facilities, which are based on the self-help therapy of the Alcoholics Anonymous twelve recovery steps.

METHADONE MAINTENANCE

Methadone, a legally controlled synthetic medication that produces little, if any, high, yet relieves craving and withdrawal symptoms, is used to assist in withdrawal from heroin.

NONMETHADONE OUTPATIENT TREATMENT

Drug counseling and therapy or medications other than methadone are used to treat marijuana, or psychedelic or multidrug users to reduce cravings.

RESIDENTIAL TREATMENT CENTERS

Staffed by both formerly chemically dependent persons and professionals, therapeutic communities are designed to foster behavioral and personality changes in patients in order for them to learn to live without drugs.

269. COMMON INFORMATION PROVIDED ON OVER-THE-COUNTER DRUG LABELS

➡ Name and address of the manufacturer, distributor, or packer

➡ Lot, control, or batch number

➡ Name of the product

➡ Type of drug

➡ Active ingredients

➡ Symptoms or conditions for which the product should be used (indications for use)

➡ Warnings and cautionary statements (i.e., who should not be taking the drug, adverse reactions that could develop from use, symptoms that signal the need to see a doctor, how long the drug should be taken, etc.)

➡ Precautions about interaction with other over-the-counter drugs and alcohol

➡ Directions for proper and safe use

➡ The expiration date (month and year beyond which the product should not be used)

➡ Patent number

➡ Any special offers from the manufacturer

➡ Any special instructions for package opening or handling

➡ Price of the product

➡ UPC (Universal Product Code) symbol

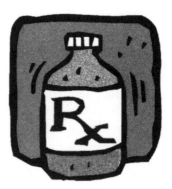

270. UNITED STATES DRUG LAWS

THE FEDERAL FOOD, DRUG, AND COSMETIC ACT (1938)

➡ Outlaws the sale of impure and falsely labeled drugs

➡ Requires manufacturers to prove to the FDA that a new drug is safe before they sell it

➡ Requires that drug labels list active ingredients, directions for use, and warnings of possible harmful effects

THE DRUG AMENDMENTS ACT (1962)

➡ Requires drug companies to prove that a new product is effective and safe

COMPREHENSIVE DRUG ABUSE PREVENTION AND CONTROL ACT (THE CONTROLLED SUBSTANCES ACT—1970)

➡ Laws governing manufacture, use, sales and distribution of illicit drugs

FDA REGULATIONS (1975)

➡ Ensures that all trade-named and generic equivalents of the same drug have identical actions in the body

FDA REGULATIONS (1978)

➡ Requires that the labels of all prescription drugs and most nonprescription drugs carry an expiration date to show how long the drug will remain fully effective

THE ORPHAN DRUG ACT (1983)

➡ Encourages drug manufacturers in the United States to work with new drugs that can be used in the treatment of rare diseases

➡ Includes regulations that help reduce the expenses of developing and marketing orphan drugs (drugs that pharmaceutical firms cannot afford to develop)

➡ Provides federal grants to pay for some of the costs of research and development

THE FEDERAL ANTI-TAMPERING ACT (1983)

➡ Prohibits tampering with containers or labels for foods, drugs, or cosmetics

271. SOURCES OF SUBSTANCE ABUSE PREVENTION EDUCATION AND INFORMATION

AL-ANON FAMILY GROUPS
(212)-302-7240
Al-Anon/Alateen
http://www.Al-Anon-Alateen.org
For an Al-Anon or Alateen meeting near you in Canada or the U.S., dial 1-800-344-2666

NATIONAL ASSOCIATION FOR CHILDREN OF ALCOHOLICS
11426 Rockville Pike, Suite 100
Rockville, Md 20852
1-888-554-2627
http://www.health.org/nacoa

THE NATIONAL CLEARINGHOUSE FOR ALCOHOL & DRUG INFORMATION
P.O. Box 2345
Rockville, MD 20847-2345
1-800-729-6686
http://www.health.org

NATIONAL MENTAL HEALTH SERVICES KNOWLEDGE EXCHANGE NETWORK
1-800-789-2647
http://www.mentalhealth.org

NATIONAL INSTITUTE ON DRUG ABUSE (NIDA)
5600 Fishers Lane, Room 10-05
Rockville, MD 20857
301-443-6480
http://www.nida.nih.gov

PENNSYLVANIA LIQUOR CONTROL BOARD
Bureau of Alcohol Education
Northwest Office Bldg., Room 602
Harrisburg, PA 17124-0001
717-772-1432

U.S. DEPARTMENT OF EDUCATION
National Library of Education
600 Independence Avenue, SW
Washington, D.C. 20202-0498
1-800-424-1616
http://www.ed.gov/

AGING, DEATH, DYING, AND SUICIDE

272. PHYSICAL CHANGES DUE TO AGING

VISIBLE CHANGES:

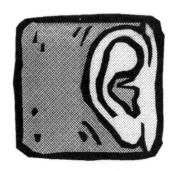

➡ Less lean body mass
➡ More fat tissue
➡ Thinning hair; loss of natural hair color
➡ Wrinkled skin (due to less elasticity)
➡ Brittle nails

OTHER CHANGES:

➡ Slower heart rate (as heart becomes less efficient in pumping blood)
➡ Impaired vision
➡ Impaired hearing
➡ Weakened muscular strength
➡ Brittle bones (because of gradual calcium loss)
➡ Reduced body energy (due to body's diminishing ability to use glucose)
➡ Less efficient immune system
➡ Less efficient endocrine system (secretes fewer amounts of hormones)
➡ Stiff joints
➡ Weakened vital capacity (measured by total amount of air from lungs that a person can exhale after a deep breath)
➡ Slower kidney functions
➡ Slowing down of basic metabolism

273. MAJOR CONCERNS OF THE ELDERLY

CRIME	Many of the elderly become housebound because they fear physical danger and loss of valuables.
RETIREMENT	Financial burdens and psychological adjustments inherent during retirement are a major concern.
NURSING HOMES	The possible need to be institutionalized is a major concern of the elderly because of the often publicized abuses, such as patient neglect.

274. MYTHS ASSOCIATED WITH THE AGING

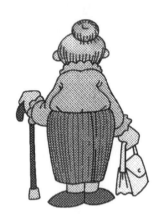

OLD AGE IS A DISEASE

➡ Old age is neither a physical nor emotional illness, but a normal process of life

MOST OF THE AGING POPULATION IS BEDRIDDEN AND DEPENDENT

➡ In truth, most elderly people are self-sufficient

ALL OLDER PEOPLE ARE THE SAME

➡ The elderly have as markedly different lifestyles and characteristics as do young people

PHYSICAL AND EMOTIONAL LIMITATIONS IMPLY AN INABILITY IN FUNCTIONING

➡ Most of the elderly cope well with difficulties, including retirement, death of a spouse, and physical limitations

THE ELDERLY ARE NOT INTERESTED IN SEX

➡ Sexual desire and activities continue well into old age, depending on physical health and cultural beliefs

275. REASONS FOR STUDYING DEATH AND DYING

➡ To understand the meaning of the word death and the legal, moral, and ethical aspects that must be considered

➡ To plan for one's own death or a loved one's death by preparing wills, funeral arrangements, and burial

➡ To understand the cultural and historical perspectives of death, and how they differ in other countries and at other times in history

➡ To help cope with the prospect of one's own death and the death of loved ones

➡ To understand how a dying person should be treated

➡ To foster a healthy outlook on death in order to better focus on life

276. CONDITIONS NECESSARY TO DETERMINE DEATH

The Harvard Ad Hoc Committee of Harvard physicians, philosophers, theologians, and lawyers judged a person to be dead if the following conditions existed over a 24-hour period:

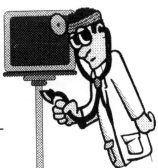

➠ Unreceptivity and unresponsivity—pertains to a total lack of awareness of external stimuli; irreversible coma

➠ Lack of reflex movements—fixed and dilated pupils, no response to bright light, no central nervous system activity

➠ Flat electroencephalogram—no electrical brain activity as indicated by this test

➠ Lack of movement and breathing—no muscular or respiratory movement during one hour of observation by a physician

277. DEFINITIONS OF DEATH

➠ Biological Death—occurs when all parts of the brain have died, although organs may still be alive and may be transplanted to another person

➠ Brain Death—involves an absence of electrical activity of the brain as indicated by an electroencephalogram

➠ Cardiac Death—refers to a stoppage of the beating of the heart

➠ Cellular Death—occurs when the body cells die over a period of hours or days

➠ Legal Death—occurs when the death certificate is signed

➠ Somatic Death—refers to the sudden death of the body, such as that which may occur in an automobile accident

278. LEADING CAUSES OF DEATH

LEADING CAUSES OF DEATH IN THE UNITED STATES:

➡ Heart Disease

➡ Cancer

➡ Stroke

➡ Accidents

LEADING CAUSES OF DEATH (15- TO 24-YEAR-OLDS)

➡ Accidents

➡ Murders

➡ Suicide

➡ Cancer

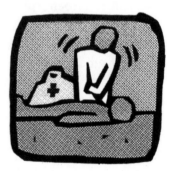

279. FACTORS THAT DETERMINE OUR ATTITUDES ABOUT DEATH

Personal experience	Family values
Religious beliefs	Knowledge
Family attitudes	Emotions
Cultural views	Age

280. DEVELOPMENT OF A CHILD'S UNDERSTANDING OF DEATH

AGES 2–5   Death is recognized but not understood as being permanent. Death may be viewed as sleep.

AGES 5–9   Death is beginning to be recognized as being permanent, but there is an inability to understand it as something that could happen to them. Death may be personified as an angel, skeleton and so on.

BY AGE 10   Death is viewed as being permanent, irreversible, and inevitable. Inability exists to understand that it can happen to anyone at anytime.

281. STAGES IN THE ACCEPTANCE OF DEATH

According to Elisabeth Kubler-Ross, the five stages in the acceptance of death are:

DENIAL   Iinitial reaction to any loss, that is often accompanied by feelings of isolation and loss.

ANGER   Ocurs when the victim can no longer deny his or her illness or loss.

BARGAINING   May involve praying, seeking alternative treatments, or promising better behavior in exchange for the death.

DEPRESSION   Involves a period of grieving for the loss; the situation is sad and the person has the right to be depressed.

ACCEPTANCE   Involves a coming to terms with the situation without feelings of hostility; allows time for facing reality in a constructive way.

282. DEFENSE MECHANISMS USED TO COPE WITH DEATH

By using the following coping devices, people dealing with death and dying are better able to unconsciously protect themselves from threatening situations.

FANTASIZING   By imagining certain solutions or outcomes, individuals are able to work through many of the problems that may be of concern to them.

IDENTIFICATION   An individual can gain a sense of belonging and self-worth by identifying with other people.

PROJECTION   Individuals may blame something or someone for their own failure or shortcoming.

RATIONALIZATION Individuals may deceive themselves in order to cope with a failure or disappointment by rationalizing the situation to fit their needs.

REGRESSION   An individual desires to get rid of the tensions and return to the carefree days of his or her youth.

REPRESSION   An individual may exclude painful experiences, impulses, or fears from his or her mind.

SUBSTITUTION   An individual may replace one goal with another in order to gain self-respect.

283. COMMON STRATEGIES USED TO COPE WITH DEATH

It is only natural to experience grief when a loved one dies. The National Mental Health Association suggests the following ways to cope effectively with the pain:

➡ Seek out caring people. Find friends and relatives who can understand your feelings of loss or join support groups with others who are experiencing similar losses.

➡ Express your feelings. Tell others how you are feeling; it will help you to work through the grieving process.

➡ Take care of your health. Maintain regular contact with your family physician and be sure to eat well and get plenty of rest.

➡ Accept that life is for the living. It takes effort to begin to live again in the present and not dwell on the past.

➡ Postpone major life changes. Try to hold off on making any major changes to give yourself time to adjust to your loss.

➡ Be patient. It can take months or even years to absorb a major loss and accept your changed life.

➡ Seek outside help when necessary. If your grief seems to be too much to bear, seek professional assistance to help come to terms with your loss and work through your grief.

284. WAYS TO HELP OTHERS GRIEVE

If someone you care about has lost a loved one, you can help the person through the grieving process using the following techniques:

➡ Share the sorrow. Allow her or him to talk about feelings of loss and share memories of the deceased.

➡ Don't offer false comfort. It doesn't help the grieving person when you say "it was for the best" or "you'll get over it in time." Instead, offer a simple expression of sorrow and take time to listen.

➡ Offer practical help. Babysitting, cooking, and running errands are all ways to help someone who is in the midst of grieving.

➡ Be patient. Remember that it can take a long time to recover from a major loss. Make yourself available to talk.

➡ Encourage professional help when necessary. Don't hesitate to recommend professional help when you feel someone is experiencing too much pain to cope alone.

For further information contact:

NATIONAL MENTAL HEALTH ASSOCIATION
1021 Prince Street
Alexandria, VA 22314
Phone 800-969-6642
http://www.nmha.org

GRIEF RECOVERY INSTITUTE
8306 Wilshire Blvd.
Beverly Hills, CA 90211
Phone 800-445-4808

285. COMMON METHODS OF FINAL DISPOSITION OF A BODY AFTER DEATH

INTERMENT:

➡ The deceased is buried or interred in the earth in a cemetery or memorial park. This is the most common method.

CREMATION:

➡ The body is incinerated and reduced to ashes through intense heat—approximately 2,200°. The remaining residue is commonly called "ashes" but has more weight than ashes and is of a consistency resembling gravel. The remains are usually scattered, buried, or placed in an urn or other container.

ENTOMBMENT:

➡ The casket containing the body is placed in an above-ground building or Mausoleum that has vaults for a number of entombed bodies.

286. PEOPLE MOST SUSCEPTIBLE TO SELF-DESTRUCTION

A person has a greater suicidal predisposition if he or she has experienced any of the following:

➠ Previous suicide attempt

➠ Previously threatened suicide—directly or indirectly

➠ Chronic illness

➠ Recent death of a loved one

➠ Financial stress
    Job loss
    Bankruptcy

➠ Domestic difficulties
    Divorce
    Separation
    Broken home

➠ Severe depression
    Feelings of hopelessness, guilt, or shame

➠ Alcoholism

➠ Drug use

➠ Family history of suicide

➠ Inability to cope with stressful situations

Many different groups are at a higher risk of committing suicide:

➠ Elderly: Elderly people, particularly those with chronic illnesses, have the highest suicide rate of any age group

➠ Adolescents/Young Adults: Suicide attempts are among the leading causes of hospital admissions in people under 35

➠ Schizophrenia: One third of people with schizophrenia attempt suicide

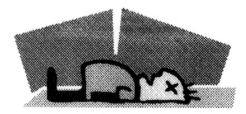

287. CAUSES OF TEEN SUICIDE

Suicide, the intended taking of one's own life, is one of the leading causes of death for people between the ages of 15 and 19. The causes of teen suicide include the following:

➟ They may have difficulty coping with who they are, where they belong, and who cares about them

➟ They may have pressures to be responsible and to succeed

➟ They may experience failures in relationships

➟ They may experience failures in school or work

➟ They may become pregnant or have a sexually transmitted infection

➟ They may get in trouble with the law

➟ They may be unable to cope with feelings of failure or loss through death or divorce

© 1999 by The Center for Applied Research in Education

288. WARNING SIGNS OF SUICIDE

Four out of five teens who attempt suicide have given clear warnings. *Pay attention to these warning signs:*

VERBAL WARNING SIGNS

➟ Direct statements, such as "I wish I were dead," "I don't want to live anymore," or "I want to die."

➟ Indirect statements, such as "They'll be sorry when I'm gone," or "I can't take it anymore."

BEHAVIORAL WARNING SIGNS

➟ Giving away possessions

➟ Frequent accidents

➟ Depression

➟ Lack of energy

➟ Increased or decreased appetite

➟ Changes in sleeping or eating patterns

➟ Withdrawal from normal activities

➟ Severe drop in school performance

➟ Increase in risk-taking activities

➟ Personality changes

➟ Previous suicide attempt

➟ Obsession with death

➟ Poems, essays, and drawings that refer to death

➟ Dramatic change in personality or appearance

➟ Irrational, bizarre behavior

SITUATIONAL WARNING SIGNS

➟ Experiencing a loss (death, divorce, etc.)

➟ Having difficulties with family

➟ Experiencing difficulties in school or at work

➟ Abusing drugs or alcohol

➟ Getting into trouble with the law

➟ Having no significant other person in their lives

➟ Experiencing low self-esteem due to failure

289. SUGGESTIONS FOR HANDLING POTENTIAL SUICIDES

➡ If a person threatens suicide, take him or her seriously

➡ Ask whether the person has a specific plan and means to follow through with it

➡ Be direct; talk openly and freely

➡ Allow the person to express his or her feelings

➡ Do not give advice

➡ Express what you think, but do not be judgmental

➡ Do not dare or challenge the person

➡ Do not allow yourself to be sworn to secrecy

➡ Be willing to listen. This affirms a person's feelings.

➡ Suggest to the person that he or she call a suicide center or crisis intervention center, or talk with a trusted teacher, counselor, doctor, member of the clergy, or other adult. If the person refuses, talk to one of these people or your parents for advice on handling the situation.

NATIONAL MENTAL HEALTH ASSOCIATION
1021 Prince Street
Alexandria, VA 22314-3615
Phone 800-969-6642
http://www.nmha.org

AMERICAN ACADEMY FOR CHILD
AND ADOLESCENT PSYCHIATRY
Wisconsin Avenue, NW
Washington, DC 20016
Phone 800-333-7636

AMERICAN ASSOCIATION OF SUICIDOLOGY
4201 Connecticut Avenue, NW
Suite 310
Washington, DC 20008
Phone 202-237-2280

290. INDIRECT FORMS OF SELF-DESTRUCTION

Some people find life intolerable and unmanageable, and participate in death-oriented behaviors, such as

Overeating	Accidents
Overworking	Alcoholism
Heavy smoking	Careless driving

291. MYTHS ABOUT SUICIDE

MENTIONING SUICIDE MAY GIVE A PERSON THE IDEA

➡ Suicidal people already have the idea. Talking about suicide openly and freely can help to prevent a person from acting on the idea.

ALL SUICIDAL PERSONS ARE MENTALLY ILL

➡ Although the suicidal person may be extremely unhappy and upset, he or she is not necessarily mentally ill

ONCE PEOPLE ARE SUICIDAL, THEY ARE BEYOND HELP

➡ The suicidal crisis lasts only for a limited amount of time. The person can get help and improve.

IT'S NOT A SUICIDE IF THERE IS NO SUICIDE NOTE

➡ Only about one in four suicide victims leave notes